# CONFLICT AND CONTROL
## IN
## HEALTH CARE ADMINISTRATION

Volume 14, Sage Library of Social Research

# SAGE LIBRARY OF SOCIAL RESEARCH

# Conflict and Control in Health Care Administration

**Jerry L. Weaver**

Foreword by MILTON I. ROEMER

Volume 14
SAGE LIBRARY OF
SOCIAL RESEARCH

SAGE PUBLICATIONS      Beverly Hills      London

*For information address:*

SAGE PUBLICATIONS, INC.
275 South Beverly Drive
Beverly Hills, California 90212

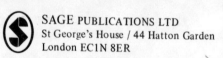

SAGE PUBLICATIONS LTD
St George's House / 44 Hatton Garden
London EC1N 8ER

Printed in the United States of America

International Standard Book Number 0-8039-0447-9(P)
0-8039-0448-7(C)
Library of Congress Catalog Card No. 74-82998

FIRST PRINTING

*For*
*Rocky, Sherrie, and Maura*

# TABLE OF CONTENTS

# FOREWORD

This is a book about administration of health service, mainly in hospitals, grounded in organization theory and built upon a body of empirical data. The data were collected from interviews with a sample of administrators of institutions and agencies in Southern California; they were interpreted in the light of the author's background as a political scientist, well versed in the field of organizational dynamics.

But this small volume is more than a report of a field research project. It is a vivid account of the background of current health administrators, the problems they face and the skills they must have. It enlightens us, therefore, about the current issues of health administration in an increasingly complex world of health services.

In the long history of medicine, or the healing arts, health administration is a newcomer. Small wonder that it has its problems, both with patients and with the diversity of health personnel providing direct patient care. It is the complexities of health service organizations, of course, that have created the need for administrators; yet most of the personal health care providers involved in those organizations have barely come to accept their roles in a social setting. The training, the traditions, the values of doctors and nurses emphasize a one-to-one relationship between the healer and the patient. Other factors, like the social demands of teamwork, the hierarchical requirements of organizations, the realities of financial or quality controls are regarded at best as necessary evils, if not as positive irritants.

Administration, therefore, requires sophistication not only about the workings of organizations but also about the behavior of people, especially people under stress. Professor Weaver's initial motivation in undertaking this study was to learn something about the type and content of education needed to help students acquire that sophistication. And it is not surprising to find that the responses of health administrators to questions about what they think they need to know coincide so well with the author's theoretical analysis of what they *ought* to know. It is mainly the social sciences and management tools; to a lesser extent, medical needs and technology.

Perhaps this may help to explain Professor Weaver's finding that hospital administrators are, on the whole, conservative. That is, they see their role as conserving or protecting the institution, working for its survival against forces that might weaken or destroy it—forces from within or without. They see their task as maintaining stability.

Put in another way, they are emotionally inclined not to rock the boat, or to try to stop others from rocking the boat, lest it capsize. Yet this attitude, while understandable, creates a paradox in the world of health service. For the very essence of the medical sciences is constant advancement, and a central feature of democratic society is rising expectations or demands for the benefits of that advancement. Hence, the administrator who craves stability may often find himself crushed in the middle between the technical and social forces for change and the organizational compulsives for tranquillity.

Perhaps the task is to educate health administrators in the strategy of the gyroscope, which keeps the ship moving forward on an even keel in a stormy sea. Easier said than done, of course. The job turnover among hospital administrators, as Professor Weaver reports, is high, because few of them have mastered this strategy. Yet, real progress in the organized health services comes from the leadership of those few who have.

In America, more than other nations, the tasks of the health administrator are tough. Our technological advancements are especially great, yet our tradition for individual freedom is particularly strong; in other words, Americans want the benefits of technology but often resist the organizational measures required to apply it. Years ago William Ogburn described this as "cultural lag." In countries with stronger social or collective traditions, the task is less difficult—and small wonder that in Great Britain or Sweden, the Soviet Union or Yugoslavia, the professional tenure of health administrators is longer.

In the American hospital, more than other types of health service entity, the battle lines between organizational requirements and the individualistic ideology are sharply drawn. Our hospitals are typically "open staff." The private attending doctor's first commitment and devotion are to his private practice and his private patient—only secondarily to the hospital organization. Of course, this is changing as medical staff structuring becomes more rigorous. The more highly structured health care organization may present the administrator a bigger job but a less frustrating one.

Perhaps if more public health or community health administrators had been included in Professor Weaver's research sample, the resultant portrait would be somewhat different. In the general community, the weight of forces against professional individualism are usually greater than inside the four walls of a hospital. Not that conflicts at the community level are lacking, but if countervailing pressures are mobilized, movement forward is possible without collapse of the system.

It is this dynamics which has led many of us engaged in educating hospital administrators to insist that they be taught a good deal about unmet community health needs, the relevance of which to "running a facility" may not be immediately apparent. Only through knowledge of such needs will the administration of a hospital or other health facility be inspired to be innovative, although this means rocking the boat and perhaps even losing his job. In the long run, conflicts in the social organization of the health services have been followed by progress.

It is encouraging that in the 1970s Professor Weaver finds

career mobility occurring mainly within the health services. This is in contrast to my own studies of over 15 years ago, when most administrators had come into the world of health service from other origins. The point is that formal training of nonphysicians in health service administration is relatively recent. Yet, because the need has grown so steadily, the educational programs in health and hospital administration have expanded rapidly. With this, the demands of health institutions and agencies to have trained administrators have continually risen, and the numbers of professional health administrators have, of course, enlarged.

Today there is in America a growing corps of educated and, let us hope, increasingly sophisticated and courageous health administrators. It is on their shoulders that must fall much of the task of providing leadership to improve the nation's health services, to make them more responsive to total human needs. Education for achieving "control" requires knowledge of the social sciences and managerial techniques that Professor Weaver's study has elaborated. But it also requires appreciation of the inevitability of "conflict," which this study has also underscored. Thus, it is both conflict and control that characterize health administration today.

From the conflict there can emerge progress, but only if it is guided constructively. The health administrator thus gains control of the situation, rather than becoming discouraged or frustrated. This, as I see it, is the important lesson that Professor Weaver's book can teach.

–Milton I. Roemer, M.D.
*Professor of Health
Services Administration
University of California
Los Angeles*

# PREFACE

This study reports the findings of a survey of the activities and problems of a cross section of health care administrators from various types and sizes of institutions. A model of health care administration was employed which stresses the central function of the administrator to be the extraction and allocation of resources: economic goods and services, information, legitimacy, prestige, and coercion. These resources are required for the survival of the institution and are held by individuals or bodies called *sectors*. These sectors are found both within and outside of the health institution. It is the task of the health administrator to form ongoing relationships (structures) with these sectors and to negotiate and facilitate the exchange of the institution's resources for those of the sectors. The particular individuals or bodies with which the administrator interacts are called *role partners*. Because the different role partners and other individuals with which the administrator interacts have alternative expectations for the behavior of the administrator, the administrator's behavior becomes the subject of conflict—the struggle by role partners and others to enforce their expectations and demands by manipulating the resources they control to sanction the administrator.

This structural-functional orientation to the role of the health administrator places him in the context of supporting and maintaining the institution. In this regard, the model is essentially conservative: we shall view the effects of administrative behavior not as it bears of the provision of "good" or "progressive" services, but only as it relates to the survival of the institution in its given state.

This was done in order to underline the significant position the administrator holds in the system of health care which exists in the United States. By emphasizing the resource exchange role of the administrator, we place his responsibilities for the operations and quality of the institution squarely in a central place—a centrality that is often overlooked by analyses which conceptualize the administrator as a part of the health delivery team or as a member with physicians, nurses, and other members of the health industry of a social hierarchy. It is my view and contention that the potential power and actual responsibility of the administrator are great and need to be clearly understood as resting on the dynamic created by every bureaucratic organization: the need to exchange resources with other bureaucratic institutions in order to survive. It is in the context of organizational theory, not health care or medical sociology, that the administrator should be viewed. Our resource exchange and role expectation model of administration offers such an insight.

The design of this research was largely completed before I saw Wolf Heydebrand's powerful and provocative *Hospital Bureaucracy: A Comparative Study of Organizations.* His work covers the organizational context within which the administrator operates and is the source of many hypotheses about the relative impact on organizational behavior of size, occupational and departmental specialization, and type of administrative structure. While I have attempted to introduce facets of his research to the present discussion, no *ad hoc* treatment can do justice to the significance of Heydebrand's research. His volume should be read in concert with the present one.

This research was made possible by a grant from the Center for Health Manpower Education, California State University, Long Beach. I deeply appreciate the help and understanding of Professor J. J. Thompson and Ms. Margaret Taylor of the Center. The following is the better for the criticism and suggestions of Ms. Barbara DePaola.

*—Long Beach, California*

*Chapter 1*

# PROFILE OF THE PROFESSIONAL
# HEALTH CARE ADMINISTRATOR

Among the changes and innovations that have occurred in the health care industry since 1945, none has been more pronounced than the rise of the nonmedical professional health care administrator. The health care administrator plays a major part in planning, organizing and supervising the diverse activities encountered in all types of health care delivery institutions. Typically, the full-time, nonclinically trained administrator sees that the patient's records are properly kept, the patient is fed, the physical plant is maintained in good order, and the resources the hospital, clinic, or medical center requires to provide its services are available. It is not an overstatement of his activities to say that the administrator shares responsibility with the medical staff for the care and treatment provided by the facility.

These and other tasks which comprise health care administration are not a new dimension of the provision of care;

indeed, the solo practitioner who takes time to balance his accounts or the managing partner of a small proprietary hospital who dictates a letter ordering supplies is engaged in administrative activities. What is new, however, is the emergence of the health care administrator as a separate professional stratum within the health care industry. Several factors are related to this appearance. With the growing technical complexity of medicine and the concomitant proliferation of specializations has come the physical concentration of services in such organizations as group practices, prepaid medical programs, medical centers, extended care facilities, and the like. Here the range of supportive services is so extensive as to require full-time supervision and coordination. But more is involved than simply giving full-time attention— the financial, personnel, records management, dietetic, housekeeping and community relations tasks required to support complex health care organizations require skills and experiences not provided by clinical education.[1]

Recent legislation and court decisions have imposed numerous and complex regulations and restrictions on health care providers. These conditions must be adhered to in order to raise funds, protect the facility against law suits, and handle withholding and social security tax records of employees. For example, federal programs such as Medicare and Medicaid have changing reimbursement formulae and eligibility standards which require continuous attention, experience in completing forms, and an eye for administrative bargaining as well as an awareness of political, economic, sociological and judicial precedents and trends. Any facility desiring federal funds is required to submit elaborate budgetary proposals, progress reports, and pounds of supporting paperwork. Nor is the expanding role of the federal government alone responsible for the bureaucratization of the health care system. The rise of third party payment (i.e., health and medical insurance programs) brought in its wake reporting and record-management requirements of a huge magnitude and vast scope.[2]

Another force which has moved the industry toward professional administrators is the growing unwillingness to "waste" medically-trained personnel in essentially administrative duties when trained administrators are available. The post-1945 expansion of public education has brought forth increasing numbers of individuals schooled in business administration, social sciences, and other disciplines who possess formal training in personnel, finance, records, community relations, organization and methods, and other administrative specialties. As these graduates have entered the field of health care administration, they have sought to protect and advance their claims of professional competence; thus from the beachhead established by the nonmedically trained administrators during the 1950s has come pressures for the recognition of the professional stature of the new arrivals. To a considerable extent, these efforts have been successful—associations, journals, college specializations, and accreditation procedures bear witness to the drive for "professional" status.[3]

Aside from the forces and innovations within the industry that have brought forth organizational and procedural complexity, the rise of the professional administrator is partially the result of the prevailing bureaucratic nature of the social institutions with which health care facilities must do business. For example, the dramatic post-1945 expansion of the health insurance industry, the rise of federal agencies which disburse grant monies, the growth of large, operationally complex networks of supply providers, the organization of most of the industry's personnel in one form or another of collective bargaining agency, and, most recently, the creation of planning and coordinating boards and agencies are bureaucratic enterprises with which health care facilities now must interact. Thus the evolving organizational complexity of the health industry is both a reaction to and a stimulus for the bureaucratization of other social institutions.[4]

None of these forces is declining—technology continues to grow at an exponential rate, eligibility formulae change, new programs are offered by the government, and alternative forms of delivery—such as free clinics, health maintenance organizations, mobile outreach programs—multiply. Universities and colleges are redirecting their resources to meet the anticipated personnel demands of the health industry; and the federal government is establishing various regional and comprehensive health planning programs that demand elaborate information from and sophisticated collaboration of all types of health care facilities. Thus, there is good reason to assume the continued expansion both in numbers and tasks of health care administrators.

Who is this creature, the health care administrator? Where does he come from? What does he do? Where is he going? The answers to these and other questions should be pondered by students of health care delivery, analysts of the behavior of client-centered service bureaucracies, teachers of would-be administrators, and practicing health care administrators.

This book summarizes answers to these questions found in a study of administrative personnel from 46 health care facilities in a metropolitan region of Southern California. The range of institutions was intentionally broad: short-term acute care hospitals, extended care institutions, a Veterans Administration facility, free clinics, convalescent hospitals, county medical centers, small proprietary hospitals, and health maintenance organizations (see Table 1). Rated bed capacity ranged to nearly 2,000. Interviews were obtained from chief administrative officers, their administrative assistants, and department administrators. Chiefs of medical staff were not interviewed. However, in some cases, the head of the nursing staff was interviewed because the facility's policy opened this position to an individual other than a nurse. A total of 111 completed interviews was obtained: 17 administrators of convalescent hospitals, 22 chief administrative officers of short term and extended care institutions, 43 department administrators, 23 administrative assistants (and associate or assistant hospital administrators), and 6 directors or administrators of outpatient clinics.

Table 1

Composition of Sample by Type of Facility[1]

| Type of Facility | Number of Facilities Contacted | Permission Received | Interviews Obtained |
|---|---|---|---|
| Proprietary Convalescent Hospitals | 31 | 16 | 17 |
| Proprietary Acute Care Hospitals | 7 | 3 | 3 |
| Proprietary (Industrial) Clinics | 1 | 1 | 1 |
| Nonprofit Acute Care Hospitals | 10 | 10 | 35 |
| Nonprofit Health Maintenance Organization (Different Locations) | 3 | 3 | 14 |
| Nonprofit Clinics | 5 | 5 | 5 |
| Nonprofit Alcohol Hospitals | 1 | 1 | 1 |
| County Hospitals | 4 | 4 | 20 |
| District Hospitals | 2 | 1 | 1 |
| State Mental Hospitals | 1 | 1 | 3 |
| Veteran's Administration Hospitals | 1 | 1 | 11 |

[1] Based on designations supplied by State of California, Department of Public Health, Hospitals, Nursing Homes and Related Health Facilities Licensed by the State of California (Sacramento: Bureau of Health Facilities Licensing and Certification, 31 March 1972).

Each interview was conducted in private by a graduate student from a health care administration program. The questionnaire included both open-ended and structured items and obtained basic biographic information (age, sex, education, career pattern, etc.), a profile of how the administrator spent an average working day, and the administrator's description of the major problems or tasks with which he had to deal. To chart the territory covered by administrators, an open-ended question ("What are the main tasks or problems you have to handle?") was complemented by a series of direct queries ("Is determining costs of patient services and care a major problem? Do professional and staff organizations and unions cause you any particular problems?" etc.). One aim of the research was to fill the void noted by Rychlin, Pointer and Levey in data regarding career channels, patterns of professional development, and the functional tasks of administration in the health field.[5]


## "He is a College-Educated Anglo"

A man and his son are driving down a freeway when their car is involved in a major accident. The man is killed; the badly injured boy is rushed to a nearby hospital. As the boy is being prepared for surgery, the attending physician glances across the room at him. "Oh my God! My son, my son," cries the doctor.

The resolution of this apparent contradiction—as anyone familiar with the feminist movement knows—is that the physician is the boy's *mother.* The infrequency of encountering female physicians (in the United States) gives the story its mystifying (and pointed) twist.[6]

In the context of the present research, "administrator" could justifiably be substituted for "physician": only 24% of the sample is female. But even this disproportion is not evenly distributed, either across the various types of facilities or within the administrative hierarchy. As Table 2 indicates, women are found as department heads (usually in housekeeping, dietetics and nursing) in large nonprofit "voluntary" hospitals. They are very nearly excluded from senior administrative positions in large institutions: only 13% of all chief administrative officers are women. As has been reported by other researchers, women are restricted in health care administration to a narrow range of positions while being largely excluded from offices of central authority.[7]

Considering the fact that all the facilities covered in the research are located in a multiethnic area, one containing large populations of Asians, Blacks, and Chicanos, it is striking that among the 111 respondents interviewed we encountered only four Blacks, one Asian, and no Chicanos. Of these minority administrators, *all* were found in government facilities. The under-representation of ethnic minorities (including women) is doubtless the consequence of a number of factors: the relatively few members of these communities who receive college training in the disciplines from which administrators are recruited; the competition for "qualified"

Table 2

Distribution of Female Respondents

by Type of Facility and Occupational

Category

| Type | Percent of Sample | N |
|------|------------------|---|
| Proprietary | 22.2 | 6 |
| Nonprofit | 55.6 | 15 |
| Government | 22.2 | 6 |

| Occupation | Percent of Sample | N |
|------------|------------------|---|
| Convalescent Hospital Administrator | 22.2 | 6 |
| Chief Administrator Short Term and Extended Care Hospitals | 11.1 | 3 |
| Department Administrator | 59.3 | 16 |
| Administrative Assistant | 3.7 | 1 |
| Outpatient Clinic Administrator | 3.7 | 1 |

minority members from other employers; and overt and implicit discrimination in hiring and promoting. The under-representation of minorities (and the improbable distribution of women) in health administration calls for close examination and speedy remedial action.

The composite Anglo male administrator has at least one college degree: only 23% of the sample reports no college degree. Moreover, the chances are good that he holds a Master's degree: one-third of the sample does. However, there is quite an array of academic specializations counted among the respondents. No fewer than thirty-five different under-graduate majors were reported. Business administration accounted for fifteen individuals, with accounting and nursing nine each, psychology seven, and economics six. Other fields include sociology, public administration and English (four individuals each), political science, history, and geography (three each), and military science (one). Among post-graduate specializations, hospital administration (fifteen) was the most common, followed by business administration, public health, and social work/welfare (five each). It is clear that the graduates of the approximately 30 hospital administration and health care administration programs form only a tiny fraction of the practicing health care administrators. While there is increased (and increasing) awareness of these professional programs, and emphasis on finding recruits from them to fill administrative posts, one's identity as a health care administrator is as much self-conferred as academically determined. Even among the younger, more recent entrants into the profession, there is no appreciable shift toward business, public, or health care administration training. Apparently, health care facilities hire individuals, not degrees.

## Career Patterns

Each respondent was asked to list all of the jobs or positions he had held since leaving school. These responses were coded so as to reveal the extent to which individuals moved into the health administration field vertically or horizontally—that is, entered administration and continued to their present position or came to this position from outside the industry. Table 3 summarizes the career patterns.

Table 3

Career Pattern Prior to Present Position

| Previous Employment | Percent of Sample |
|---|---|
| Health Administration Only | 45.9 |
| Patient Care, Nonadministration | 2.7 |
| Administration, Public Sector | 7.2 |
| Administration, Private Sector | 6.3 |
| Neither Health nor Administration | 2.7 |
| Mixed with Some Previous Health Administration | 29.8 |
| First Job | 5.4 |
| Total Number of Cases | 111 |

As we see, very few middle and top level administrators are without previous administrative experience. For almost one-half of the individuals sampled health care administration has been their only career. This finding suggests a good deal of vertical mobility within the industry. Discounting those whose present job is their first since entering the labor force, only 13.5% of the sample have moved horizontally into health administration from non-health industry employees. Overall, about three out of ten report cross mobility—moving back and forth between health administration and other occupations. It is noteworthy that very few current administrators (2.7%) moved into their positions from the medical and nursing staffs or other nonadministrative occupations within the health care industry. Apparently the once common practice of physicians becoming administrators is no longer followed: only three of the respondents report holding the M.D. degree.

Combining the career patterns with the data regarding academic preparation, we speculate that the facilities recruit on the basis of likely potential for advancement, and then train upper level staff through what amounts to an apprentice program—starting administrators in subordinate positions and then promoting those who demonstrate aptitude. Such a system could produce a rapid turnover as superior individuals are promoted, undesirable ones fired, and marginal cases moved out of the mainline slots used to season candidates for advancement.

Indeed, such a pattern is suggested by the data on length of tenure in present position. In the overall sample, 27.9% report holding their present positions 12 months or less; almost the same proportion (26.1%) report tenures of over five years (see Table 7). While the extreme frequency of turnover may be accounted for by the dynamic expansion of opportunities for employment as new facilities are built and others expanded, I suspect that the apprentice-like up-or-out approach is also responsible.

The relatively high turnover and rapid mobility of personnel, plus the apparent absence of specific educational prerequisites for recruitment, suggest an answer to the question about the administrator's origins. As we saw, he comes to his present position from college by way of other health administration jobs. Another dimension of where he comes from, using the expression "where he comes from" in the colloquial sense of motives and goals, is suggested in the answers to the question: "Why did you choose to work at this particular facility?" Over 15% replied that the position represented either a promotion or an increase in salary (or both). But 27.9% said that the present position offered them an opportunity to develop their own ideas about how a program should be run; offered more freedom, challenge, or responsibility; was of more professional interest; provided an opportunity to work in a dynamic, modern or otherwise stimulating facility. Common to these responses is the theme of greater *professional* satisfaction.

## Professional Involvement

There is considerable literature dealing with the emergence of health administration as a professional identity. Most of the commentators deal with the struggle for recognition, status, and power between administrators and physicians.[8] The conflict between administrators and physicians is the result of a number of factors and is played out in a complex set of structural relationships we shall examine below. Here it suffices to establish that administrators have been successful in establishing a professional identity, if not in completely resolving their status inequities vis-a-vis physicians. A visible force in this development has been the professional association (such as the American College of Hospital Administration, American Hospital Association, and such regional associations as the California Association of Hospital Administrators). These organizations have created a focus on and have given expression to health care administration.[9]

Associations provide workshops, in-service training, and

other educational activities for members—programs widely mentioned by the respondents as important sources of information about and solutions for current professional problems. In addition, the associations publish periodicals geared to the practical day-to-day situations, current trends, and new developments faced by administrators. Scanning through issues of *Hospital Topics, Hospitals, Hospital Progress* and the more specialized publications such as *Hospital Financial Management* reveals not only articles and news of interest to administrators, but also a wide variety of advertising that brings to their attention new products and services.

Accordingly, it seems reasonable to conclude that professional associations and periodicals are focal points for professional interest. Heydebrand found that among chief administrative officers of teaching hospitals, a type of health care facility he (and other analysts) labels "the elite" of the industry, the median number of professional association memberships was four, compared with a median number of memberships in nonprofessional organizations (civic, church, recreational and social, political) of only one.[10] Following from our discussion and this finding, we hypothesize that membership in professional associations and reading professional periodicals is a reliable indicator of professional interest. Moreover, the relationship between involvement and membership and reading is direct: an increase in cumulative memberships/reading of periodicals indicates increased involvement with health care administration as a profession.

In order to index the strength of the sample's identification with health administration, we created a measure of identification by combining the respondent's reported number of professional association memberships and journals "regularly" read. Table 4 presents a summary of the rank order distribution of the sample.

Without rankings on appropriate indices of professional involvement of firemen, CPAs and aerospace engineers, it is impossible to assess the present sample's relative level of

Table 4

Index of Professional Involvement

| Professional Involvement Index | (Score) | Percent of Sample |
|---|---|---|
| Neither belongs to an association nor reads a journal | (0) | 0 |
| Reads 1 or 2 journals or holds membership in 1 or 2 associations | (1) | 5.4 |
| Reads 3 or more journals or holds 3 or more memberships | (2) | 18.9 |
| 3 or more memberships (or journals) plus 1 membership (or 1 journal); 1 or 2 journals plus 1 or 2 memberships | (3) | 26.1 |
| 1 or 2 journals (or memberships) plus 3 or more memberships (or journals) | (4) | 31.6 |
| 3 or more journals plus 3 or more memberships | (5) | 18.0 |
| Total Number of Cases | | 111 |

professional involvement. And while the present sample does not equal the median four memberships reported by Heydebrand, it is remarkable that nearly half of the sample placed in the upper end of the index by reading three or more journals (or holding three or more memberships) *and* belonging to one or more associations (or reading one or more periodicals).

## Trends

Thus far we have discussed our findings in relative isolation: figures have been presented as one dimensional phenomena set down in a single time frame, and therefore devoid of any continuity, insensitive to the historical forces that have given rise to them and within which they have no social significance. Are administrative cadres growing more representative of the overall population? Are there discernible trends in educational preparation? Career mobility? Are there more or fewer women and ethnic minorities among today's administrators?

Answering questions about trends and patterns is tricky business. Longitudinal analysis (that is, studying a given phenomenon at successive points in time) requires rigorous controls so that we can be reasonably sure that what variation (or lack of it) we find is the consequence of whatever independent variable we may be studying, and not of asking different questions to different samples or similar methodological errors. In order to check for trends or patterns in the health care profession, we should apply the same questions to as similar a set of facilities as possible at regular intervals.

If we apply this rigorous standard of methodological purity, then no longitudinal analysis is possible. But if we are willing to forego rigor, and to bear in mind the tentative nature of the findings, a suggestive analysis is possible. Although they vary greatly in sample composition, data gathering techniques, and the universe from which respondents were drawn, several previous studies of health care administrators are available from which we can draw selected demographic data to compare with those generated by the present study.

Table 5 provides some evidence for speculating about trends. We see that the presence of women and ethnic minorities in health care administration has remained a largely constant and disproportionately small fraction, although perhaps there has been a slight increase recently in the representation of the former.

Educational preparation shows little basic change: roughly the same percent of all samples possess a post-graduate college degree. The variation in percent reporting no college degree very likely reflects the differential composition of the samples. Depending on the geographic distribution, type and size of facilities from which respondents were drawn, we

Table 5

Summary of Selected Characteristics from Studies of Health Care Administrators

| Characteristic | Roemer[1] | Elling & Shepard[2] | Dolson[3] | Heydebrand[4] | Weaver |
|---|---|---|---|---|---|
| Sex | | 12.7% Female | 21% Female | | 24.3% Female |
| Ethnicity | | 2.0% Black | | | 3.6% Black<br>.9% Asian |
| Education | 6% w/o degree<br>14% BA<br>35% advanced degree in Pub Health or Hosp., Adm. | 14.4% w/o degree | 28% w/o degree<br><br>43% advanced degree | 31% some academic training in Hosp. Adm. | 23.4% w/o degree<br>17.1% BA<br>34.2% advanced degree |
| | 42% MDs | | 12% MDs | | 2.7% MDs |
| Careers | 26% previous health adm experience | 83.3% previous health adm experience | | 84% previous health adm experience | 76.5% previous health adm experience |
| Tenure in Present Job | | | 50% less than 6 years | 6 yrs median tenure | 27.9% 1 yr or less |
| Year data Gathered | 1958 | 1964 | 1965 | NA | 1973 |
| Total Number of Cases | 428 | 7976 | 4038 | 791 | 111 |

1
Milton I. Roemer, <u>Medical Care Administration: Context, Positions, and Training in the United States</u> (San Francisco: American Public Health Association, Western Branch, 1963), 86-88A.

2
Ray H. Elling and William P. Shepard, "A Study of Public Health Careers: Hospital Administrators in Public Health," <u>American Journal of Public Health</u>, 58(1968), 918-924.

3
Miriam Dolson, "Where Women Stand in Administration," <u>Modern Hospital</u>, 108(1967), 100-105; and Mirian Dolson, Rodney F. White and Paul Van Ripper, "Study Reveals What Administrators Earn," <u>Modern Hospital</u>, 106(1966), 103-106.

4
Wolf V. Heydebrand, <u>Hospital Bureaucracy: A Comparative Study of Organizations</u> (New York: Dunellen, 1973), 196-197.

would expect a rather wide variation in educational background. Personnel from small rural facilities in the South and Midwest repeatedly report much lower educational attainment levels than their peers in large facilities on either coast.

I do think it significant, however, that we observe a steady and marked decline in the percent of M.D.s among health care administrators. This datum is bolstered by other accounts that indicate that this is a major trend across the country during the past decade.

Except for Roemer's pioneering study, there is a continuing pattern of recruiting individuals with previous health care administration experience. From what I can see in the other studies, this pattern may be somewhat misleading because of the exclusion of middle level occupations. These studies, national in scope, have usually dealt only with chief administrative officers, individuals who normally are health administration careerists. In the present study, we include other administrative positions: department head, administrative assistant, clinic administrator. If we exclude these respondents and deal only with chief administrative officers of short term and extended care hospitals, the figure reporting previous administrative experience climbs to 95.5%. Whichever way we figure it, it is clear that health care administration positions continue to be filled from within the health care administration profession and that the route to the top is a ladder, not a boarding plank.

The two most recent national studies (Dolson's and Heydebrand's) indicate a fair degree of occupational stability: typically, administrators had served about six years in their position when interviewed. In the present study, only 26.1% reported tenure of *five* years or longer; the median tenure is approximately two years. As we see from Table 5, nearly three in ten reported tenure of one year or less. The very rapidly expanding job market for health care administrators, especially in Southern California, plus the fact that many of the facilities in the sample are less than five years old, probably affect the present tenure profile. But since similar forces have been at play in other parts of the country, spurred by the Hill-Burton hospital construction project, population shifts, and general concern across the country about providing better health care, I suspect that the median tenure of all levels of health care administrators nation-wide has dropped over the past five or so years.

Looking at the aggregate profiles of the health care administrators, we see emerging a picture of an Anglo male college graduate who has remained in health administration since securing his first position in the profession. He has a high level identification with the profession which finds expression in his willingness to change jobs, and often employers, to find challenging, stimulating, and professionally rewarding opportunities, or to become associated with prestigious institutions or individuals. This professionalism is also illustrated by his joining several professional associations and reading several trade periodicals.

In the context of previous studies of health administrators, we see that there may be a slightly greater percent of women among the present sample; surely there are fewer M.D.s. The present sample, especially the top administrators, continues the pattern of vertical mobility; however, the duration of the present sample in its current position is much shorter than the previously reported median length of tenure.

# NOTES

1. W. V. Heydebrand, *Hospital Bureaucracy: A Comparative Study of Organizations* (New York: Dunellen, 1973), 195.

2. Cf., A. R. Somers, *Hospital Regulation: The Dilemma of Public Policy* (Princeton: Princeton University, Industrial Relations Section, 1969).

3. J. R. Griffith, "An Educational Challenge for the Programs and the Practitioners: The New Role of the Administrator," *Hospital Administration* 12 (1967), 127-142.

4. R. N. Wilson, "The Physician's Changing Hospital Role," *Human Organization* 18 (1959-1960), 179.

5. H. S. Ruchlin, D. D. Pointer, and S. Level, "Health Administration Manpower Research: A Critique and a Proposal," *Hospital Administration* 18 (1973), 91-92.

6. Although clothed in lacy social science jargon, Croog's observation is perhaps a little less obscure to those aware of sexism: "The relations of female doctors with their male peers, with subordinate workers, and with patients are complicated by relative importance of female status as opposed to professional status." S. H. Croog and D. F. Ver Steeg, "The Hospital as a Social System," in H. E. Freeman, S. Levine, and L. B. Reeder (eds.) *Handbook of Medical Sociology*, 2nd. ed. (Englewood Cliffs, N.J.: Prentice-Hall, 1972), 287. Also see J. J. Williams, "Patients and Prejudice: Lay Attitudes toward Women Physi-

cians," *American Journal of Sociology* 51 (1946), 283-287; Ibid., "The Woman Physician's Dilemma," *Journal of Social Issues* 6 (1950), 38-44; P. H. Beshiri, *The Woman Doctor: Her Career in Modern Medicine* (New York: Cowles, 1969); E. Lutker, *Women Gain a Place in Medicine* (New York: McGraw-Hill, 1969); B. Ehrenreich and D. English, *Witches, Midwives and Nurses: A History of Women Healers* (Old Westbury, N.Y.: The Feminist Press, 1972).

7. Cf., M. Dolson, "Where Women Stand in Administration," *Modern Hospital* 108 (1967), 100-105.

8. E. M. Lentz, "Hospital Administration—One of a Species," *Administrative Science Quarterly* 1 (1957), 444-463; H. L. Wilensky, "Dynamics of Professionalism: The Case of Hospital Administration," *Hospital Administration* 7 (1962), 6-25.

9. M. I. Roemer, "Education for Medical Care Administration," *Hospital Administration* 10 (1965), 6-18.

10. Heydebrand, *Hospital Bureaucracy,* 198.

*Chapter 2*

# OCCUPATIONAL VARIATIONS

One of the central aims of this research is to explore the career patterns and professional problems of health care administrators. So far we have grouped all the respondents in the sample and treated their profiles monolithically. Yet this collective approach hides a good deal of what we wish to reveal: the existence of variations in profiles and patterns within the profession. We are told by previous research that the personnel and work routines of proprietary hospitals differ from those of government facilities;[1] there are differences between administrators of extended care institutions such as mental hospitals and those of short term facilities;[2] and there are differences according to rated bed capacity.[3] Accordingly, we shall look closely at the influence of the type, size and services provided by our respondents' institutions to see if these situational conditions of employment are associated with career and professional differences.

Aside from variations associated with size, type of service and other structural dimensions of health care, there is the functional component; that is, variations associated with the administrator's assignment or occupational specialization.[4] Occupational variations among health administrators are pronounced because of the vast array of services and tasks associated with the provision of health care. Some of the variations parallel the type of service provided; for example, the duties and routines of convalescent hospital administrators differ markedly from those of their colleagues in specialized clinics; and extended care facility administrators have tasks associated with the custodial aspects of patient maintenance that are absent in the milieu of short term facility administrators. But the principal determinant of occupational variation is the wide range of technical, clinical, and supportive services found within most health care facilities.[5] Hospitals, extended care and short term alike, are characterized by hierarchically structured administrative systems that reflect the organization of tasks in relatively specialized units.[6] Typically, hospitals (and health maintenance organizations [HMOs] as well as multifunction clinics) are organized into departments—dietetics, housekeeping, medical records, nursing, maintenance, community relations, personnel, finance and planning, and so on. Above the operational level, coordination and direction is vested in several offices beneath the chief administrative officer; these intermediate offices are often charged with planning and development, operations, or finance. This intermediate administrator, responsible for supervising several departments or interrelated services or operations, may be called associate or assistant administrator, or (as in this study) administrative assistant.[7]

Administrative personnel vary not only in terms of the breadth of tasks for which they are responsible, but also according to degree and content of specialization. In the present analysis, we shall examine career profiles and professional problems associated with five occupational categories:

convalescent hospital administrator, chief administrative officer of an extended care or short term hospital, department administrator, administrative assistant, and out-patient clinic administrator. (Personnel from HMOs have been integrated into their generic category; for example, HMO department administrators are grouped with department administrators, hospital administrators with chief administrative officers, and so forth.) First, we shall scan the biographic profiles of the five categories to determine the similarities and differences among them in such matters as age, education, sex, tenure, professional identification, and career patterns. Once we have established this background information, we shall be prepared to analyze the variations that exist in how the categories spend their time, the major problems they see themselves dealing with, and the sources of their problems. In order to highlight the comparisons, we shall introduce the selected characteristics serially and point out the intercategorial variations.

In the following discussion, references to the clinic administrator category is omitted. The limited number of respondents in this group (six) precludes meaningful analysis. I feel that the under-representation of this group is a major lacuna because this particular form of health care provision is expanding dramatically. Part of this expansion is represented by the free clinic movement that sprang up in the late 1960s and continues to increase. In the Southern California area, for example, where there was one free clinic in 1967, there are 49 in 1973. Other clinics, such as neighborhood health centers, venereal disease and pregnancy problem centers, crisis centers, alcohol and drug centers, are increasingly found in urban areas. Moreover, the rapid growth of prepaid health maintenance programs (HMOs) has spawned more outpatient clinics. Another aspect of the significance of clinic administration is the specialized services they typically provide, often to rather specialized clientele. Thus recent and rapid expansion of this sector of the industry, plus the nature of the services and clients involved, may very well produce a cluster of administrative problems that are unique to this type of facility. The clinic administrator deserves far more attention than we are able to give him. In hopes of stimulating further study of clinic administrators, we shall include data from this category in the following tables.

## Age

Table 6 reveals that chief administrative officers (CAOs) as a group are older than department administrators (DAs) or administrative assistants (AAs). Convalescent hospital administrators follow the age profile of CAOs. Apparently seniority is the operative principal in staffing the more complex and responsible positions. Since we have found that previous health administration experience is nearly universally associated with top administrative personnel (see Table 5), it fol-

Table 6

Age Profile by Occupational Category

| Age at Last Birthday | Convalescent Hospital Adm | Chief Adm Short Term & Extended Care Hospital | Department Adm | Administrative Assistant | Outpatient Clinic Adm | Total Sample |
|---|---|---|---|---|---|---|
| Less than 30 | 17.6 | 0 | 16.3 | 17.4 | 16.6 | 14.5 |
| 30 - 35 | 23.5 | 4.5 | 18.6 | 39.1 | 16.7 | 20.7 |
| 36 - 40 | 0 | 22.7 | 11.6 | 8.7 | 0 | 10.8 |
| 41 - 45 | 5.9 | 18.2 | 14.0 | 4.3 | 16.7 | 11.7 |
| 46 - 50 | 23.5 | 13.6 | 11.6 | 8.7 | 0 | 12.6 |
| 51 - 55 | 17.6 | 27.3 | 16.3 | 4.3 | 0 | 15.3 |
| over 55 | 11.8 | 13.6 | 11.7 | 13.0 | 50.0 | 14.4 |
| Total Number Of Cases | 17 | 22 | 43 | 23 | 6 | 111 |

lows that such experience would tend to be associated with advanced age. Note that Table 6 shows the presence of numerous 35 and younger AAs (56.5% of the category); this datum, along with the relative seniority of the CAO group, suggests that individuals are recruited on the basis of potential, either from outside the institution or promoted from the technical or production ranks, and then are advanced to other positions—for instance, are made DAs if they demonstrate capacity for administration. The U-shaped distribution curve of convalescent administrators, with 41.1% of the group 35 and younger, 0% 36 to 40, 5.9% 41 to 45, and 29.4% over 50, suggests a somewhat different pattern. Several of the younger convalescent administrators, in response to the question "Why did you choose to work at this particular hospital?" indicated that their parents or another family member owned the institution. I suspect that the privileges of proprietary control are largely responsible for many of the younger convalescent administrators—after all, Henry Ford II spent very little time working on the assembly lines of Ford Motors Corporation.

## Tenure in Present Position

We noted above that the present sample has a markedly lower median length of tenure in present position than has been reported for other groups of health administrators. Table 7 demonstrates that short tenure is common across the occupational categories. Bearing in mind that some variation results from small subsamples that form the units of analysis, there are no significant differences.

While the dynamic quality of the profession, with frequent changes of job and possibly employer, may be viewed as a boon to the ambitious mobile individual, rapid turnover may be disruptive of administrative routine and therefore dysfunctional for the quality of health care service provided.[8]

Communication and coordination break down because it takes middle level administrators time to adjust to the par-

Table 7

Length of Tenure in Present Position by Occupational Category

| Time In Present Position | Convalescent Hospital Adm | Chief Adm Short Term & Extended Care Hospital | Department Adm | Administrative Assistant | Outpatient Clinic Adm | Total Sample |
|---|---|---|---|---|---|---|
| Less than 6 months | 11.8 | 4.5 | 7.0 | 8.7 | 0 | 7.2 |
| 6 to 12 months | 17.6 | 27.3 | 11.6 | 30.4 | 33.3 | 20.7 |
| 1 yr, 1 day - 3 yrs | 29.4 | 22.7 | 37.2 | 30.4 | 33.3 | 31.5 |
| 3 yrs, 1 day - 5 yrs | 23.5 | 13.6 | 11.6 | 17.4 | 0 | 14.4 |
| 5 yrs, 1 day - 7 yrs | 5.9 | 18.2 | 14.0 | 4.3 | 0 | 10.8 |
| more than 7 yrs | 11.8 | 13.6 | 18.6 | 8.7 | 33.3 | 15.3 |
| Total Number of Cases | 17 | 22 | 43 | 23 | 6 | 111 |

ticularities of their new positions, to establish rapport with their peers, and to determine the operational (informal) expectations of the institution, its clients, and its community. Similarly, subordinates need time to confirm the expectations and work rhythm of their superiors. Certainly, the ramifications of frequent personnel changes vary with the position involved. Turnover at a junior administrative assistant post will have little overall impact on the operations of the facility. But when the head of a major department or a chief administrative officer is replaced, considerable time may be wasted, opportunities missed, and resources unwisely spent while the settling-in process takes place. For the roughly 30% of institutions in which CAOs and convalescent hospital administrators report a year or less service in their present positions, turnover may constitute a major problem, the ramifications of which are not easily seen.

This is not to suggest that personnel turnover in the middle and upper ranks has a totally or even largely negative consequence. The new men bring previous experience, mature judgment, and often skills and expertise beyond those of their predecessors. Moreover, if the notions we have about the causes of high turnover and mobility are correct, there is very little likelihood that the pattern will be drastically altered in the present decade. New facilities will be opened, existing ones expanded, and competition for jobs from graduates of health administration programs will spur turnover. Nevertheless, the impact of administrative personnel turnover on the health care industry—especially from the point of view of the delivery of patient services—bears close and further analysis.

Perhaps an indication of some of the consequences of rapid personnel mobility may be glimped by looking at the past 10 years in the history of higher education in the United States. During the 1960s the academic community experienced the booming growth and easy mobility that apparently characterizes today's health industry. Some universities opted to build and strengthen their programs by recruiting mid-career, seasoned professionals (i.e., associate professors). Others went after superstars and raided back and forth for senior scholars. Openings for junior faculty increased rapidly with many departments doubling their size in five or six years. Positions were filled with bodies: Ph.D.s from second and third level institutions were easily employed; ABDs from prestigious national and major regional schools were fast to be recruited.

This rapid growth and expansion was accompanied shortly with mass student unrest, demands for radically new student-professor and professor-administrator relationships, and a dramatic withdrawal of public confidence in and financial support for higher education. Faculties unionized, students marched, administrators resigned (or died or were fired), and legislatures refused to appropriate money. Clearly, growth and mobility were not solely, perhaps not even significantly, responsible for the massive disruptions and changes in the academic community. But the two phenomena are associated in time and place. Students of the health care delivery industry might do well to ponder the apparent similarities of their field at the present time with academia ten years ago; such a comparison could suggest how to avoid the negative and encourage the positive consequences realized during the period by higher education.

### Academic Preparation

While convalescent hospital administrators are also businessmen who must deal with a wide range of operational problems, they differ markedly in educational preparation or previous work experience from other health care administrators. Convalescent hospital administrators report fewer post-graduate programs of study, especially when compared with chief administrative officers. But as Table 8 illustrates, both categories are about equally as likely to have been administration or business majors in college.

Department administrators and administrative assistants are noticeably higher than CAOs and convalescent hospital administrators in the frequency with which they report a social science background. Why the high percent (21.6% in the total sample) of social science graduates? Is this because of the increased numbers of social science graduates in the job market? That is, are there proportionately more social science graduates being hired now than 10 or 15 years ago? The data suggest not: approximately as many older respondents as younger ones reported social science majors.

It may be, then, that the higher percent of social science majors among DAs and AAs is merely due to a sampling error; if we had interviewed 500 CAOs, DAs and AAs, we

Table 8

College Preparation by Occupational Category

| Major or Area of Concentration | Convalescent Hospital Adm | | Chief Adm Short Term & Extended Care Hospital | | Department Adm | | Administrative Assistant | | Outpatient Clinic Adm | | Total Sample | |
|---|---|---|---|---|---|---|---|---|---|---|---|---|
| | Undergrad | Grad | Undergrad | Grad | Undergrad | Grad | Undergrad | Grad | Undergrad | Grad | Undergrad | Grad |
| No College | 17.6 | 76.5 | 4.5 | 27.3 | 4.7 | 39.5 | 13.0 | 26.1 | 0 | 50.0 | 9.9 | 41.4 |
| Public or Business Administration, Management | 29.4 | 0 | 36.4 | 54.5 | 18.6 | 30.2 | 13.0 | 52.2 | 16.7 | 0 | 22.5 | 33.3 |
| Accounting, Finance Operations Research, "Business" | 5.9 | 5.9 | 27.3 | 0 | 16.3 | 4.7 | 17.4 | 0 | 16.7 | 16.7 | 17.1 | 3.6 |
| Biology, Zoology, Health Sciences | 11.8 | 5.9 | 22.7 | 9.1 | 18.6 | 7.0 | 17.4 | 8.7 | 16.7 | 16.7 | 18.0 | 8.1 |
| Sociology, History, Psychology, Social Sciences | 11.8 | 5.9 | 9.1 | 4.5 | 25.6 | 9.3 | 30.4 | 13.0 | 33.3 | 16.7 | 21.6 | 9.0 |
| Other | 17.6 | 5.9 | 0 | 4.5 | 14.0 | 7.0 | 8.7 | 0 | 16.7 | 0 | 10.8 | 4.5 |
| Total Number of Cases | 17 | | 22 | | 43 | | 23 | | 6 | | 111 | |

might have come up with equal frequencies of social science majors in each category.

Alternatively, it may be that many institutions have a policy of filling certain positions with individuals who have sociology, social welfare, social psychology, political science or public administration backgrounds. With the rise of community relations, comprehensive health planning, new governmental funding and reimbursement programs, collective bargaining and grievance procedures with staff unions and associations, and other essentially social and political dimensions in the health institution's environment, it makes good sense to hire individuals with related backgrounds and experience to complement the clinical, technical and managerial specialties among the administrative cadre. The National Commission on Community Health Services declared: "Special emphasis must be given to securing and preparing top-level health service administrators for responsible positions of leadership in health. This will entail selective recruitment and training that includes administrative management, economics, sociology, and political science."[9] Looking to the interests of the institution in its battle for economic, social, and political support, Raffel argues that "the effective health administrator must be able to talk the language of the government officials, the legislators, the fiscal experts, and the public if he wishes to be heard, understood, and to get his way."[10] He concludes that a social science background is an optimal preparation for "getting his way."

## Previous Health Administration Experience

In light of the notion that convalescent hospitals are administered by businessmen rather than professional health administrators, the findings reported in Table 9 come as somewhat of a surprise. Apparently convalescent hospital administrators have not moved over from shoe stores, ice cream parlors, or insurance offices; rather, they come to their

Table 9

Career Prior to Present Position by Occupational Category

| Previous Employment | Convalescent Hospital Adm | Chief Adm Short Term & Extended Care Hospital | Department Adm | Administrative Assistant | Outpatient Clinic Adm | Total Sample |
|---|---|---|---|---|---|---|
| Health Adm Only | 41.2 | 63.6 | 46.5 | 39.1 | 16.7 | 45.9 |
| Health Adm & nonhealth Administration | 41.2 | 31.8 | 23.3 | 34.8 | 50.0 | 31.5 |
| Nonhealth Adm Only | 5.9 | 4.5 | 20.9 | 13.0 | 0 | 12.6 |
| No Previous Adm Exper. | 11.8 | 0 | 9.3 | 13.0 | 33.3 | 9.9 |
| Total Number of Cases | 17 | 22 | 43 | 23 | 6 | 111 |

present position, just as other health care administrators, from within the industry. If there is a significant characteristic of convalescent hospital administrators, it is that they largely have remained in the convalescent sector while few administrators of short term and extended care facilities have had experience there.

It appears that convalescent hospital administration may be a rather specialized occupation which recruits from within its own domain and, perhaps, places less emphasis on educational degrees and training (e.g., compared with the other categories nearly three times as many of this category report no post-graduate education—Table 8).[11] If this pattern is a matter of choice and not one of inability to compete with other types of facilities for the available trained administrators, then note should be made.[12] The number of convalescent hospitals will increase greatly over the next decade; in part because of the growing number of Americans who live longer, in part because government and private insurance programs make institutional care (rather than retention in the family or maintenance in public institutions) financially within the reach of more and more elderly persons, and in part because it may be a very profitable enterprise for investors.

## Professional Involvement

If, as I have suggested, convalescent hospital administrators constitute a discernable sector within the health care industry, this separate task/identity structure could explain the markedly lower professional involvement scores reported by Table 10. Ten times as many convalescent administrators as CAOs fall in the lower end of the involvement scale. Even this score profile is somewhat misleading. Typically, respondents in the other categories reported memberships in the American College of Hospital Administration, American Hospital Association, and the Hospital Council of Southern California. They read *Hospitals, Modern Hospital, Hospital Administration,* and *Hospital Topics.* Convalescent administrators, however, report few memberships in these associations and little reading of the aforementioned journals. Instead, the memberships and readings that built their index scores include the American College of Nursing Home Administrators, California Association of Nursing Homes, American Nursing Home Associates, *Modern Nursing Home,* and *Nursing Homes.*

Allowing for the relatively small numbers in each category and the sample error that could produce variations of many percentage points, the concentration of the chief administrative officers at the high end of the professionalism scale is noteworthy. Again, this variation might be accounted for by the disproportionately greater number of older men in the CAO category. The reasoning is that men who have just entered the profession would have had less time or opportunity to become aware of the rewards from association memberships and journal reading. But Table 11 scotches this

Table 10

Ranking on Professional Involvement Scale by Occupational Category

| Prof. Involvement Scale | Convalescent Hospital Adm | Chief Adm Short Term & Extended Care Hospital | Department Adm | Administrative Assistant | Outpatient Clinic Adm | Total Sample |
|---|---|---|---|---|---|---|
| 1 Point (low) | 5.9 | 4.5 | 4.7 | 4.3 | 16.7 | 5.4 |
| 2 Points | 35.3 | 0 | 16.3 | 21.7 | 50.0 | 18.9 |
| 3 Points | 35.3 | 9.1 | 34.9 | 21.7 | 16.7 | 26.1 |
| 4 Points | 17.6 | 50.0 | 27.9 | 39.1 | 0 | 31.5 |
| 5 Points (high) | 5.9 | 36.4 | 16.3 | 13.0 | 16.7 | 18.0 |
| Total Number of Cases | 17 | 22 | 43 | 23 | 6 | 111 |

Table 11

Ranking on Professional Involvement Scale by Age

| Professional Involvement Score | Age at Last Birthday | | | | | | | |
| | Less than 30 years | 30-35 | 36-40 | 41-45 | 46-50 | 51-55 | Over 55 | Total Sample |
|---|---|---|---|---|---|---|---|---|
| 1 (low) | 13.3 | 4.3 | 0 | 0 | 7.1 | 5.9 | 6.2 | 5.4 |
| 2 | 33.3 | 26.1 | 8.3 | 7.7 | 21.4 | 17.6 | 12.5 | 18.9 |
| 3 | 6.7 | 30.4 | 41.7 | 46.2 | 28.6 | 17.6 | 18.8 | 26.1 |
| 4 | 40.0 | 26.1 | 25.0 | 38.5 | 14.3 | 35.3 | 43.7 | 31.5 |
| 5 (high) | 6.7 | 13.0 | 25.0 | 7.7 | 28.6 | 23.5 | 18.8 | 18.0 |
| Total Number of Cases | 16 | 23 | 12 | 13 | 14 | 17 | 16 | 111 |

speculation. Except for the youngest segment of the sample, scores do not vary significantly by age. Because age is the only biographic variable in which the CAO category differs appreciably from the others, the finding that age has little effect on index scores lends support to the idea that CAOs are a highly committed group who, along with meeting their institutional, community, and personal obligations, maintain a distinctively high level of involvement with the vehicles of their profession.

## Professional Associations as Reference Groups

But professional associations are more than purveyors of advice and information. They are also *reference groups:* formal organizations that manifest expectations about how an adherent is to act.[13]  These expectations are either internalized (that is, become part of the cognitive and evaluate structure of the actor) or used as standards of comparison in determining the "objective correctness" of an attitude, opinion, or behavior.[14]  Membership in an association, or the occupancy of a position such as health administrator that is the object of attention by an association, is not sufficient to establish the fact that a particular association fulfills the part of reference group. Only when an individual takes on the expectations of the group in setting and judging his own norms and behavior according to those of the group does the organization become a reference group. Furthermore, actors may objectively be members of an organization (such as an administrator who belongs to the American College of Hospital Administration), yet not count this organization among his reference groups. On the other hand, the *absence* of formal membership does not preclude an organization being a major source of role expectations.

Often when we speak of "professionalization" we are implicitly recognizing the efforts of professional associations, academic programs, and prestigious individuals to establish a given set of role expectations as authoritative for a particular

occupational group. Reading the pages of the trade periodicals aimed at health administrators (or the organs of any
other occupational group) reveals how "correct" standards
are articulated to the selected audience. Such a review also
reveals that there are alternative, sometimes conflicting, sets
of expectations advanced. For example, periodicals contain
arguments in favor of the administrator playing a greatly
expanded role in determining community health needs and
marshalling resources to achieve community goals; other
commentators caution that expanded community involvement will bring the administrator into conflicts over priorities
and policies, thus politicizing the administrator and embroiling
him and his institution in essentially political (although non-
partisan) struggles.

Aside from the alternative, even contradictory, expectations emanating from professional associations, demands are
placed on the administrator because the individual who is an
administrator is also the incumbent in other social offices:
friend, family member, citizen, church member, member of
social and recreational groups. Each of these incumbencies
has multiple expectations associated with it; and since it is
difficult to determine with certainty which hat is being worn
at a particular time, expectations associated with other activities crowd in upon the individual when he attempts to
exercise his responsibilities as an administrator. Friends
call him to gain special favors in the facility; marital difficulties cause him to forego his duties in order to re-
assure his wife of his attention; religious principles intrude
into the consideration of supporting an abortion clinic
expansion.

From the perspective of role theory, the health administrator is tied into a complex web of conflicting expectations
which arise from different sociopsychological levels: the
family, the community, the organization, the society, the
professional reference group.[15] Riggs' concept of poly-
normativism describes this condition in which an actor is
faced with, and has not consistently resolved, conflicting role

expectations.[16]   In seeking understanding of the behavior of health administrators, professional associations offer important clues into the sources and resolutions of these conflicting demands that characterize the administrator's work situation.

## Department Administrators: A Comparison

In *The Community Hospital,* Georgopoulos and Mann present limited biographic data from department administrators of ten Michigan hospitals. Table 12 offers a gross comparison of the Michigan and Southern California groups. The lower proportion of women among the Southern California sample, although there are probably more women in the overall sample than would be found in a national study of top administrators (see Table 5), suggests an expression of the underlying tradition of sexism in hospitals—women are relegated to lower paying, less prestigious institutions.

A close look at the facilities covered by Georgopoulos and Mann reveals that they are medium-sized facilities (averaging 196 beds) located in nonmetropolitan areas. None of the facilities is an "elite" institution. While half of the Michigan DAs reportedly were satisfied with their salaries, no indication is made of the relative standing of their pay vis-a-vis the overall industry. We can speculate, however, that department administrators in such institutions would not be among the most highly paid element of all DAs in 1957 in the United States.

On the other hand, the Southern California DAs are drawn from large nonprofit and government hospitals with teaching affiliations (i.e., "elite" institutions according to Heydebrand), located in a metropolitan region continuing a large pool of potential administrators. One of the facilities is the nation's largest Veterans Administration hospital. Another (a nonprofit "community" hospital) has been recognized by major trade publications as an outstanding leader in the organization and delivery of health care.

Table 12

Comparison of Selected Characteristics of Two Groups of

Department Administrators

| Characteristic | Percent of Sample | |
| --- | --- | --- |
| | Michigan[1] Hospitals | Southern California Hospitals |
| Female | 58 | 37.2 |
| 40 years & older | 31 | 48.9 |
| College degree(s) | 40 | 81.4 |
| 5 years or longer with present hospital | 60 | 32.6 |
| Previous administrative experience | 33 | 69.8 |
| Data Collected | 1957 | 1973 |
| Total Number of Cases | 101 | 43 |

[1] Basil S. Georgopoulos and Floyd C. Mann, The Community Hospital (New York: Macmillan, 1962), 145.

Traditionally in the United States, women in the health industry have been disproportionately found in the less prestigious, lower paying facilities and positions.[17] Since the Michigan institutions rank well below those of California in prestige and pay (inflation of both currencies controlled), it is likely that these situational factors alone account for a great deal of the variation in the percent of the two samples that is female.[18]

Another trend that Table 12 points to is the growing emphasis on education and previous administrative experience in filling middle and upper level positions. We see that the percentages reporting college degrees and previous administrative experience have doubled between 1957 and 1973. This may indicate the increase in professionalization of health care administration. Wilensky describes the process of fashioning the mantle of expertise out of whole cloth:

> A profession claims exclusive possession of competence in a specified area. This competence is "technical" because it comes from a systematic body of knowledge acquired only through long, prescribed training. The profession represents a monopoly of skill, which is linked to standards of training and which justifies a monopoly of activity in an area. It is felt that not just anyone can do the job, so the job territory is marked "off limits" to the amateur.[19]

While knowledge and experience—and keeping amateurs off—are usually seen as favorable to the improvement of care, these same traits may have profoundly negative, and unanticipated, social consequences.

If it is true, as we have speculated, that women and ethnic minorities are relegated to less desirable facilities and positions, one result of a movement stressing recruitment and promotion based on education and experience will be to reduce the chances of women and non-Anglos securing administrative positions. When recruitment criteria are raised, it usually indicates an attempt to "upgrade" or "professionalize" a position. Almost inevitably, upgrading is associated with an increase in salary, fringe benefits and other incentives designed to attract "better people." But this now makes positions once disdained by men and therefore open to female and other disadvantaged groups, attractive. Anglo males, aside from the initial advantage they derive from the fortuitous coincidence of birth, proportionately are more highly educated and experienced. Thus Anglo males will push the less advantaged from places previously reserved for them. We have in fact seen this happen when previously Black medical schools were forced to admit applicants without regard to race. Because of their proportionately larger numbers, Anglo students won many more seats in formerly Black schools than Blacks received in formerly Anglo institutions.

Until access to education and lower level administrative positions is opened to women and non-Anglos, and until the proportion of "qualified" women and non-Anglos is significantly increased, emphasis on *achievement criteria alone* will reinforce the racial, sexual bias found in the composition of the health administration profession.

In this section we examined selected characteristics of four occupational categories of health care administrators. We found that convalescent hospital administrators differ in two respects from other categories: they are more likely not to hold a college, especially post-graduate, degree; and they are less likely to belong to professional associations or to read trade publications aimed at hospital personnel. Instead, convalescent administrators report memberships and reading of trade publications associated with the nursing home, convalescent hospital sector of the industry.

All categories of administrative personnel report high levels of previous health administration experience. And all categories are about equally comprised of persons reporting one year or less and those reporting five years and longer tenure in their present positions.

The high percents of CAOs, DAs, and AAs ranking at the upper end of the professional involvement index, especially CAOs with nearly 90% reporting two or more association memberships *and* two or more periodicals regularly read, suggest that professional associations may be important sources of behavioral and attitudinal norms for health administrators. Role theory, especially such theory that emphasizes the central position of reference groups, could prove a powerful analytical device for sorting out the complex web of demands that bear on and determine the behavior of administrators.

With the completion of this section, we have concluded our examination of the questions: Who is the health administrator? Where does he come from? In the following chapter we shall begin to develop answers to the questions: What does the administrator do? Why does he do it?

# NOTES

1. H. J. Ruchlin, D. D. Pointer, and L. L. Cannedy, "Administering Profit and Nonprofit Institutions," *Hospital Progress* 54 (1973), 67-69, 80.

2. E. Freidson, "Review Essay: Health Factories, the New Industrial Sociology," *Social Problems* 14 (1967), 493-500.

3. D. B. Starkweather, "Hospital Organizational Performance and Size," *Inquiry* 10 (1973), 10-18.

4. E. J. Connors and J. C. Hutts, "How Administrators Spend Their Day," *Hospitals* 41 (1967), 45-50, 141.

5. C. Perrow, "Hospitals: Technology, Structure, and Goals," in J. March (ed.) *Handbook of Modern Organizations* (Chicago: Rand McNally, 1965), 910-971.

6. W. V. Heydebrand, *Hospital Bureaucracy: A Comparative Study of Organizations* (New York: Dunellen, 1973); Starkweather, "Hospital Organizational Performance and Size," 10-18.

7. On the organizational hierachy, see B. S. Georgopoulos and F. C. Mann, *The Community Hospital* (New York: Macmillian, 1962).

8. S. H. Croog, "Interpersonal Relations in Medical Settings," in Freeman, Levine, and Reeder (eds.) *Handbook of Medical Sociology*, 2nd. ed. (Englewood Cliffs, N.J.: Prentice-Hall, 1972), 263.

9. National Commission on Community Health Services, *Health is a Community Affair* (Cambridge: Harvard University Press, 1966), 88-89.

10. M. W. Raffel, "Education for Health Services Administration, 1: Undergraduate Training for Health Administration," *American Journal of Public Health* 20 (1970), 984.

11. "Typical Administrator Relies on Experience, Not Classroom Work, Health, Education, and Welfare Survey Shows," *Modern Nursing Home* 28 (1972), 44.

12. See D. D. Meyers, "Practioner's View of Education for Long-Term Care Administrators," *Journal of the American College of Nursing Home Administrators* 1 (1972-73), 10-17.

13. J. L. Weaver, "Role Expectations of Latin American Bureaucrats," *Journal of Comparative Administration* 4 (1972), 133-166.

14. The function of comparative evaluation provided by reference groups is discussed by H. H. Hyman and E. Singer, *Readings in Reference Group Theory and Research* (New York: Free Press, 1968).

15. Cf., M. E. Shaw and P. R. Costanzo, *Theories of Social Psychology* (New York: McGraw-Hill, 1970), 339-342.

16. F. W. Riggs, *Administration in Developing Countries: The Theory of Prismatic Society* (Boston: Houghton Mifflin, 1964), 277, 279.

17. M. Dolson, "Where Women Stand in Administration," *Modern Hospital* 108 (1967), 100-105; *FAH Review* (symposium), "Womanpower in Hospital Administration," 5 (1972).

18. Wren reports that administrators of smaller hospitals lack the educational and experience qualifications of those in larger facilities, a finding which lends support to our claim that such individuals would be vulnerable to displacement or blocked upward mobility if an effort to upgrade their facility was undertaken. See G. R. Wren, "Administrators of Small Hospitals Have Same Motivating Factors as Those of Large, But Have Less Education and Experience," *Hospital Management* 3 (1971), 19.

19. H. L. Wilensky, "Dynamics of Professionalism: The Case of Hospital Administration," *Hospital Administration* 7 (1962), 9.

*Chapter 3*

## HOW THE ADMINISTRATOR SPENDS HIS TIME

Although there are several textbooks that tell us what health administrators *should* do, there is remarkably little systematic scientific research into what they *actually* do. How does the middle and upper level administrator spend his day? What are the typical problems and work situations he must cope with? With whom does he work? The medical staff? Patients and their families? Trustees? Personnel organizations and unions? How much of his time is spent working on financial problems? Personnel management? Preparing and reading reports? Obviously, answers to these questions offer some guidance in formulating instructional programs. If administrators spend many hours dealing with budgeting and financial matters, potential administrators should receive a firm grounding in accounting, finance, tax law, economics and the like. Similarly, courses could be provided to meet needs in personnel, records management, automated data processing, labor relations, and other areas in which administrators spend their time.

In this section we shall examine the work routine reported by our sample from two points of view: first, how the administrator spends his time; second, what he perceives to be the forces that pull him into these activities.

## Previous Research

Two studies published during the mid-1960s provide us with a point of departure as well as comparative data for our analysis. Murray, Donnelly and Threadgould analyzed the administrators of 55 Catholic acute care, voluntary hospitals and 55 non-Catholic hospitals of corresponding size and geographic location. Administrators were asked to fill out a log of all their activities on specific days between mid-November 1966 and June 1967.[1]

Connors and Hutts followed a quite different methodology. Rather than a survey research operation, they studied five administrators in a single institution.[2] The chief administrative officer, three assistant administrators and one administrative assistant of the University of Wisconsin Hospital, Madison, were observed a total of 4255 times. Using a book of random numbers to select the observation time, each administrator was checked about 34 times per day over a period of several weeks. A graduate student intruded on the administrator at the predetermined time and recorded his activities. If the administrator was alone when an observation was required, he was asked to describe the activity he was performing. (Presumably, a certain minimal amount of discretion was permitted the interviewer in interrupting the informant with such a query—at least one would hope so.) The mass of observations was categorized into six basic activities.

Table 13 presents a comparison of the two studies. Although there is slight variation in the categories of activities in the two studies, they both share the following basic scheme:

*Planning:* defining and clarifying problems, determining facts, analyzing and considering alternatives, deciding on the action to be taken and arranging for execution.

*Organizing:* dividing and grouping the work to be done, defining the established relationships between individuals filling these jobs, and assembling resources.

*Directing and Coordinating:* instruction of subordinates through proper timing and communications (i.e., staff meetings).

*Controlling:* checking and reporting of performance; may also involve taking corrective action.

*Personal tasks:* other than hospital-related activities (e.g., eating, taking calls from wife, getting a hair cut).

*Extramural tasks:* continuing education, attending institutes and meetings outside the facility, contacts with outside agencies, individuals and community groups.

Part of the discrepancies between the findings of the two studies, particularly in the "controlling" and "directing and coordinating" categories, can be attributed to variations in coding schemes. What might be "controlling" for Connors and Hutts could easily be reported as "directing and coordinating" by Murray and his associates. Additional variation stems from the disparate data-collecting process used by Connors and Hutts. While they obtained a vast number of observations, their entire study is based on five individuals from a single facility. There is no guarantee (and none is alleged by the authors) that this particular facility and respondents are in any way typical of the universe of institutions and health care administrators. Connors and Hutts doubtless have a reliable, perhaps even valid, profile of how five men in a single hospital spend their time; but they certainly do not have a sample from which we can generalize to the overall profession. Likewise, the idiosyncratic aspects of the five respondents' work routine may bias the Wisconsin profile.

Table 13

Percent of Time Hospital Administrators Spend on Various Tasks

|  | Wisconsin Administrators[1] | Catholic Hospital Adms[2] | Non-Catholic Hospital Adms[2] |
|---|---|---|---|
| Extramural | 27.6 | 22.4 | 20.9 |
| Controlling | 23.2 | 8.9 | 11.4 |
| Planning | 21.8 | 23.8 | 25.5 |
| Personal | 12.0 | 16.2 | 11.8 |
| Organizing | 7.8 | 2.9 | 3.9 |
| Directing and Coordinating | 7.8 | 24.5 | 24.6 |

[1] Edward J. Connors and Joseph C. Hutts, "How Administrators Spend Their Day," Hospitals, 41(1967), 47.

[2] Ralph T. Murray, Paul R. Donnelly and Margaret Threadgould, "How Administrators Spend Their Time: A Research Report," Hospital Progress, 49(1968), 55.

Murray and his associates use a sample of 110 hospital directors from across the country, thereby drastically reducing the risk of sampling error and, concomitantly, increasing our confidence in the validity of their findings.

But for all the computations and coefficients both studies report, it remains difficult if not impossible to tell *what* the respondents actually do. The coding schemes employed and the categories reported are so vague and imprecise as to be, for all practical purposes, meaningless. What actually do we understand from a given percentage of time spent in "planning" or "organizing?" Is there an inherent meaning in these terms that allows us to see what the individual is doing? Or allows us to comprehend the skills, techniques, and activities the person must integrate in order to accomplish it? I think not; and because of this lack of precision I have sought other means of categorizing administrative activities.

## The Administrator's Role

The process of delimiting the basic activities of the health administrator began with an attempt to conceptualize the central aspect of the administrator's function. Connors and Hutts, and Murray and his colleagues essentially see the administrator as an individual whose time is consumed doing things. To find out what is being done one needs only describe the "things."

Our approach sees the administrator as an incumbent of an office or position within an organization. Viewing the office from the perspective of the organization, we ask: What does the office of the administrator do for the organization? Our answer is that the office is the principal nexus for the exchange of resources between the organization and its environment.[3] Health care facilities must obtain money, manpower, information, legitimacy, and must defend itself from coercion or direct attack (not necessarily physical force; rather an unexpected denial of resources vital for survival at a time when survival is in question). In order to do this, the facility must pay out resources it possesses in the form of services, facilities for physicians, salaries, reports to reimbursement agencies, bills for services, and so on. It is the task of the administrative cadre to perform the exchange and allocation function.[4] This the the *role* of the health care administrator.

In carrying out his role of obtaining and allocating the resources which the facility must exchange in order to survive, the administrator plays a central part in fulfilling the facility's primary objective, which is the provision of certain health care services required by the community. Viewed from the perspective of the community, the administrator is a leader in organizing the ongoing discussion of alternative health care programs (as when the administrator participates in health care planning organizations). And the administrator is a teacher because he plays a role in informing the community about the evolving programs and needs of the health care industry as well as in providing information about health-related matters that helps citizens make personal and collective decisions about health care matters. The health care administrator is an important, perhaps the most significant, link between the organized and institutionalized delivery of health care and the community the facility serves.

In fulfilling his responsibilities to the community, the administrator must share responsibilities for the effectiveness and efficiency of patient care, both in his institution and other elements of the industry. The health care administrator must be concerned with the quality of care and the continuity of hospital-based care with other community health services: this is incumbent on him not simply as an administrator of health care but as one of the very few members of his community who possesses information about health and health care.[5] That is, when seen in his capacity as a *citizen* of a community, the individual who also happens to be an administrator is expected to place public-regard above "public relations" and "protecting the institution from liability."[6]

Here we see the possibility of the individual who is both citizen and administrator finding himself in a conflict situation. While health care facilities go to great lengths to fulfill their community responsibilities, there is always the chance that meeting the demands of the facility may place the administrator at odds with the expectations he has for himself as a good citizen. For example, the facility may own a block of houses which it plans to destroy in order to build a new wing; the residents of the houses, however, do not wish to leave—indeed, they demand that their landlord (the hospital) spend considerable funds to improve their homes. The board of directors refuses. The administrator is expected to proceed with the building program and to have the tenants evicted. But the administrator sees the plight of the tenants and, because of his notions of civic responsibility, is deeply sympathetic to their position. Which role is he to fulfill: that of administrator or that of citizen?

In the aftermath of World War II, and again during the Vietnam War, the primary obligation of the individual to follow the higher moral principle of placing duty to mankind before secular authority was stressed. The advocates of this position claim that people should be held accountable to public opinion and the law for acts which offend the dignity of mankind or which place "duty" ahead of "justice." However, knowing that he is morally right may be of little comfort to the *former* administrator who refused to sacrifice his civic principles before the alert of institutional necessity.

This discussion of the potential conflict facing the administrator when he finds the differences between the demands of his institution and the expectations of citizenship irreconcilable illustrates our previous assertion that the individual is simultaneously the incumbent in several roles. Besides administrator, the individual may be father, lover, friend, sibling, citizen, political partisan, churchman, and so forth. In reporting how the administrator spends his time, we are not concerned with activities which result from demands arising from role incumbencies other than that of his profession. While the administrator may well spend a good deal of time in these activities, they are not part of what we define as the central concern of health care administration: extracting and allocating the resources required by the facility's survival. Falling into the jargon of social science, we shall treat these activities as constituting an "intervening variable": in explaining the overall behavior of the administrator, we must take account of time spent in fulfilling other roles; but these activities do not constitute "health care administration."

## Administration As Resource Exchange

But how do we determine which interactions to observe? Surely it is not possible to make neat delimitations. Behavior may be the result of a complex set of demands and may be intended to meet expectations arising from multiple incumbencies. We have a guideline to follow when we return to our understanding of the administrative office as a component of the overall organization.

Where do the resources reside which the administrator must obtain for his facility? Conceptually, there are three distinct places or sets of resource possessors. The first is the facility itself. To some degree all institutions possess stores of money, economic goods, peoplepower, information, legitimacy, and other relatively scarce and productive commodities—the critical questions are what resources are available, how much is available, and what is the exchange value. Thus the administrator forms ongoing relationships with other actors in the facility in order to extract and allocate the resources which his subordinates, peers, and superiors control. Operationally, the offices in the health facility with which the administrator interacts include the chief of medical staff, head of nursing services, chief dietitian, board of trustees, and other section and department administrators.

A second source of resources is found with the institution's clientele. In health facilities, clients include patients, the families of patients, and affiliated physicians who come to the facility to perform their curative specialties. The organization exchanges its space, peoplepower, prestige, technical and financial recordkeeping and so forth for the cash and other resources (such as prestige associated with a famous physician) held by these clients.

The third set of resource holders are actors outside the facility such as accreditation and licensing bodies, third party payers, government agencies, community social, economic, and political elites, unions representing health workers, medical schools, and private foundations. One of the characteristics of the past decade or two has been the expansion of resources and organizations in the external environment of health facilities. Indeed, it has been the growth in this sector that has been one of the main spurs to the development of nonclinically trained health care administrative specialists.

Regardless of the incumbent, the office of health administrator, whether low or high in the hierarchy, must engage one or more of these sectors.

Following from this formulation of relationships between health care administrators and incumbents in other resource-holding offices, we can identify structural partnerships: health care administrator/subordinate, health care administrator/staff union, health care administrator/board of trustees, health care administrator/medical staff, health care administrator/patient, and so forth. Each structure can be researched through empirical observation; each administrator can be studied to see how much of his time is spent interacting with particular structural partners; each interaction can be characterized as to the basic content or method (direct, indirect; verbal, written; instructive, evaluative) involved.

In the following chapter we shall examine the administrator's work routine from the persepective of the resource-exchange conceptualization of administrative behavior. We shall look to see what tasks and what problems he becomes involved in as a result of attempting to deal with specific role partners. Following this description, we shall analyze these role partners as sources of problems for the health care administrator.

## NOTES

1. R. T. Murray, P. R. Donnelly, and M. Threadgould, "How Administrators Spend Their Time: A Research Report," *Hospital Progress* 49 (1968), 49-58.

2. E. J. Connors and J. C. Hutts, "How Administrators Spend Their Day," *Hospitals* 41 (1967), 45-50, 141.

3. See W. F. Ilchman and N. T. Uphoff, *The Political Economy of Change* (Berkeley and Los Angeles: University of California Press, 1971). An alternative formulation of an exchange theory applied to

health facilities is offered by S. Levine and P. E. White, "Exchange as a Conceptual Framework for the Study of Interorganizational Relationships," *Administrative Science Quarterly* 5 (1961), 583-601.

4. For alternative formulations of exchange theory which do not place central emphasis on resources, see P. M. Blau, *Exchange and Power in Social Life* (New York: John Wiley, 1964); G. C. Homans, *Social Behavior: Its Elementary Forms* (New York: Harcourt, Brace, 1961); Homans, "Fundamental Social Processes," in N. Smelser (ed.) *Sociology* (New York: John Wiley, 1967); and the papers by S. R. Walman, D. Easton, T. N. Clark, and T. Parsons in *Sociological Inquiry* 42 (1973).

5. The attitudes of health administrators toward the importance of various health care services vary significantly. See J. T. Gentry, et al., "Perceptual Differences of Administrators Regarding the Importance of Health Service Programs," *American Journal of Public Health* 60 (1970), 1006-1017; Gentry, et al., "Attitudes and Perceptions of Health Service Providers: Implications for Implementation and Delivery of Community Health Services." Paper presented at the 1971 annual meeting of the American Public Health Association (available from its senior author).

6. I am indebted to Professor J. T. Gentry, M.D., of the School of Public Health, University of North Carolina, Chapel Hill, for calling to my attention the interrelated nature of the administrator's civic and institutional roles and for correctly stressing the social service role of the health care facility.

*Chapter 4*

# ACTIVITY PROFILES

In analyzing the results from the questionnaires, we found that the time spent with role partners varied substantially depending on the position of the informant. Not unexpectedly, chief administrative officers and administrators of convalescent hospitals reported far more extensive interactions with external actors such as governmental agencies, accreditation bodies and community elites. Department administrators, on the other hand, spent more time with technical staff and clinical personnel (who often were their immediate subordinates).

Aside from variations attributable to occupation, the activities profiles of administrators varied both with size of facility and type of organization (that is, proprietary, non-profit or government). This latter variable was found to be associated with the type of service provided, because proprietary facilities in the present sample are almost exclusively convalescent hospitals, while most respondents from government facilities are from extended care (state mental) and Veterans Administration institutions.

Since our aim is to present an overall assessment of the four major health administration occupations found in the surveyed institutions, we have not followed the particular profiles of the specific subgroups. Rather, we have chosen to report profiles that reveal general patterns. Consequently, several tasks which involve specific role partners with specific offices within our sample (such as heads of community relations departments that spend nearly all of their time with community service groups and community elites) have been omitted because the department administrators spend little or no time with such actors. We have also compressed some activities, such as telephoning and report reading, so as to eliminate the specific object of the activity (such as calls from other members of health planning boards) because of the wide range and small degree of uniformity among administrators regarding the particular role partner (organizational, client, or external) typically involved.

## Overall Profile

Each respondent was presented with a series of administrative tasks and asked how much of his typical day was consumed by each. By far the largest percent of the overall sample's day was spent discussing work assignments or work-related problems with subordinates: 22.6% of the average day.

There are several reasons for this involvement with subordinates. Supervisors are expected to explain assignments to their subordinates, to observe their performance, and to resolve difficulties which arise in accomplishing assigned tasks. Thus, working with subordinates is generic to administration.

But there are conditions inherent in health care delivery that may be conducive to extra involvement with subordinates. Schultz and Johnson observe that "few organizations are composed of as many diverse skills as the hospital, which generally has nearly three employees for each patient and a heterogeneous health team influenced by over 300 different professional societies and associations."[1] The nature of the health facility's technologically complex work force bespeaks of the complex array of special tasks and procedures that are performed. Operational level administrators, such as department heads, are involved with their diverse and specialized employees; administrative assistants and administrative officers are required to integrate and coordinate this elaborate work force.

Apart from involvement in work problems of individual subordinates, the status barriers common to the health industry also brings administrators into interaction with subordinates. Wessen points out that communications and informal intercourse in health facilities tend to be horizontal rather than vertical. That is, members of specific occupational groups such as physicians, nurses, technicians, and attendents, tend to interact more frequently with each other than with members of the other groups. What intergroup communications that do take place are highly ritualized and formalistic—apparently there is little give and take between and among members of different groups.[2] Insofar as discussions and exchanges are inhibited, it follows that problems which might be resolved through informal give-and-take, or which might not arise if the various members of the health care team were empathic with each other, will be referred to administrators.

The overall significance of receiving, interpreting, and sending communications of various sorts is revealed by the finding that approximately one-third of the overall sample's average day is consumed preparing reports, attending staff meetings, and telephoning and handling correspondence. The place of report writing and reading in health administration is a central one. Pomrinse found that at one institution he studied a one-year count revealed that 105 separate reports were required or inspected by governmental agencies. Moreover 38 reports were made to voluntary nongovernmental agencies.[3] This is in addition to the countless single and multipage and minute- and hour-long verbal reports completed throughout the typical institution.

The overall sample spends approximately 7% of its day in *each* of the following activities: reading reports, discussing their particular responsibilities with their superiors, dealing with patients or their families, and attending to extramural activities. What is involved in the latter activity has changed somewhat over the past decade or so. Formerly extramural largely partook of interaction with other health care institutions, government agencies, or professional activities outside the institution; contemporarily, direct involvement in community activities has come to comprise a larger and larger part. Roemer suggests both the forces which have drawn the health care administrator into community activities as well as the range of this involvement in the following observation:

> The modern hospital administrator is expected to provide leadership in his community on general questions of patient-care planning, rehabilitation of the chronically ill, professional education and research, disease prevention, health insurance, service for the needy, and all the other elements of public health and medical care.[4]

The federal government has lent further impetus to community involvement by mandating, through the Comprehensive Health Planning Act, the formal representation of local health care institutions on regional medical planning boards.

Given the high percents accorded "planning" in Table 13, it is noteworthy that the present sample reported that in a typical day it spends *less than one percent* of its time reviewing existing programs with an eye to long range resource allocations, reading professional literature about new innovations in organization or programs, or thinking about future missions for the institution. In other words, the present sample spends very little time planning.

Those activities which were reported by the sample to comprise 5% or more of their average day are summarized in Table 14. The table also indicates what we have already come to realize—that there is a good deal of variation among occupational categories of health care administrators.

Table 14

Percent of Average Day Allocated to Selected Activities by Occupational Category

| Activity | Convalescent Hospital Adm | Chief Adm Short Term & Extended Care Hospital | Department Adm | Administrative Assistant | Outpatient Clinic Adm | Total Sample |
|---|---|---|---|---|---|---|
| Discussing work situation with subordinates | 20.8 | 23.6 | 23.2 | 21.6 | 11.6 | 22.6 |
| Preparing Reports | 6.3 | 8.8 | 12.9 | 12.3 | 14.0 | 11.1 |
| Attending Staff Meetings | 3.8 | 10.2 | 11.6 | 12.9 | 6.4 | 10.2 |
| Correspondence & Telephone | 10.2 | 11.0 | 9.7 | 8.7 | 13.0 | 10.1 |
| Extramural activities | 6.0 | 9.1 | 9.0 | 5.6 | 4.8 | 7.7 |
| Reading Reports | 3.8 | 7.3 | 8.3 | 10.0 | 4.2 | 7.6 |
| Discussing unit's activities w/ superior | 8.3 | 5.8 | 7.3 | 9.0 | 5.2 | 7.5 |
| Dealing w/ patients and/or their family | 22.5 | 4.0 | 3.4 | 2.4 | 18.0 | 7.1 |
| Meeting representatives of professional associations and staff organizations and unions | 9.0 | 5.6 | 5.4 | 6.9 | 5.2 | 6.4 |
| Total Number of Cases | 17 | 22 | 43 | 23 | 6 | 111 |

## Activities by Occupational Category

There are some marked similarities among the four principal categories of health care administrators. The percent of time consumed discussing operational situations with sub-ordinates is almost exactly the same across the four categories. The same may be said for correspondence and telephoning, extramural activities, and having discussions with superiors.

But we notice a distinctive profile for convalescent hospital administrators. For example, they spend five or six times more of their work day dealing with patients or the family of patients than do the three other groups. But they spend one-third as much time as CAOs, DAs and AAs attending staff meetings and reading reports. This savings seems to be largely consumed meeting representatives of staff organizations and professional associations.[5]

This distinctive profile reflects the organizational composition and service performed by convalescent hospitals. Unlike other institutions of the sample, convalescent hospitals provide little or no clinical or technical service for their patients. Rather, the patient receives what are essentially residential services: meals, recreation, personal services, and living space—services which are supportive rather than curative. Convalescent hospitals bear a strong resemblance to boarding homes; as such, they contain far fewer personnel, far less technology, and far shorter administrative hierarchies. Typically, there were only two or three supervisory personnel found in the convalescent hospitals of our sample. And these personnel tended to be operational rather than administrative; that is, a nurse given supervisory tasks, a member of the maintenance crew assigned responsibility for scheduling the shifts and seeing to it that inventories of supplies are reported to the administrator. Thus the staff management functions which consume much of the time of other administrators are reduced because there are fewer services and smaller staffs to deal with.

Because of the wide range of essentially long term care provided their clients, and the absence of alternative administrative personnel, patient problems are both more numerous and more often taken directly to the administrator. Generally, convalescent administrators are the only individuals who possess the organizational jurisdiction to which clients can turn for remedy.

The remarkable uniformity in time allocations across the three remaining principal categories of Table 14 bears comment. The percentages suggest that basically similar activities consume the short term and extended care facility administrators' time regardless of occupation. But what Table 14 does not reveal is the variation among role partners with which different groups spend their time. Superior for CAOs means the board of trustees or its equivalent. For department heads, staff meetings include the technical and clinical subordinates; for AAs, staff meetings incorporate department administrators and other middle and upper level supervisors. In meetings with his subordinates, the DA must be prepared to deal with highly technical specific problems brought up by their subordinates or peers from other departments. In conferences of supervisory personnel, DAs and AAs are more apt to discuss problems of staff management, finance, or program development. The role partners of chief administrative officers engaged in extramural activities might be the CAOs of other facilities, heads of government agencies, or representatives of private foundations. Administrative assistants or department administrators are more likely to be involved with lower level individuals on a narrower range of professional issues. For example, the personnel officer or the head of the records department meets his peers from other institutions in a topical seminar sponsored by a trade association or a would-be vendor of services or equipment.

The point is that although there is a basic similarity in what is being done, different skills and experiences are called for, depending on the particular administrative position involved.

## Size and Activities

So far we have considered only one dimension of variation among the sample of health care administrators: their occupation. There are other dimensions of health care institutions, however, that are known to be associated with behavior variations. Gentry and his colleagues report that attitudes of administrators as to what they consider important health care services and programs to be provided by hospitals vary significantly with facility size.[6] Anderson and Warkov, in an analysis of the relationship between hospital size and division of administrative responsiblity in 49 Veterans Administration and TB hospitals, conclude that "it is clear that the larger the hospital the *smaller* the percent of all personnel in administration."[7] Heydebrand's research, using elaborate controls for type of service, ownership, and division of labor within the facility, confirms the significance of size as a correlant of bureaucratization.[8]

There are essentially two operational indicators of size: the number of beds (service capacity) or the average daily patient census (actual volume of service). In the present study, we have chosen the former.

Table 15 summarizes the percent of an average day that is spent in selected tasks by administrators of different sized institutions. The column headed "no beds" contains only eight respondents, six of whom are the administrators of out-patient clinics. Again the size of this subsample precludes meaningful statistical comparison. As in the previous "occupational" tables, the "no beds" column will be reported but ignored in the discussion.

We observe that administrators of large facilities (400 beds and more) spend more of their time preparing and reading reports, and attending staff meetings than do their colleagues in smaller facilities. This suggests that communications and information dissemination problems increase with size—a logical consequence since rated bed capacity is often associated with organizational complexity, size of the adminis-

Table 15

Percent of Average Day Allocated to Selected Activities by Size of Facility

| Activity | No Beds | 1 - 99 Beds | 100-199 Beds | 200-399 Beds | 400-699 Beds | 700 & more Beds | Total Sample |
|---|---|---|---|---|---|---|---|
| Discussing work situation with Subordinates | 7.5 | 19.3 | 35.6 | 22.8 | 21.0 | 17.3 | 22.6 |
| Preparing Reports | 10.6 | 6.6 | 8.7 | 12.7 | 16.2 | 9.2 | 11.1 |
| Attending Staff Meetings | 6.5 | 6.1 | 10.4 | 9.7 | 14.5 | 10.5 | 10.2 |
| Correspondence & Telephone | 11.9 | 12.7 | 4.1 | 8.5 | 12.1 | 12.4 | 10.1 |
| Extramural Activities | 6.7 | 5.7 | 6.5 | 9.5 | 5.9 | 9.5 | 7.7 |
| Reading Reports | 3.2 | 3.4 | 7.4 | 7.5 | 9.6 | 10.2 | 7.6 |
| Discussing Unit's Activities with Superior | 3.8 | 5.8 | 12.0 | 7.0 | 6.1 | 7.5 | 7.5 |
| Dealing with Patients and/or Their Family | 13.7 | 17.0 | 9.2 | 5.3 | 0.9 | 3.6 | 7.1 |
| Meeting Representatives of Professional Associations and Staff Organizations and Unions | 3.8 | 9.3 | 6.0 | 6.0 | 2.4 | 9.5 | 6.4 |
| Total Number of Cases | 8 | 15 | 19 | 27 | 20 | 22 | 111 |

trative cadre, and number of subordinate personnel and operations to be coordinated and integrated.[9]

Administrators of the middle-sized facilities (100 to 199 beds) have a distinctive activity pattern. This category spends more of its time interacting with subordinates and superiors. Also they spend less time handling correspondence and telephoning.

The percent of time spent in staff meetings increases with size as does handling communications and report preparation and reading—that is, reflecting the growing problem of coordination and communication mentioned above. On the other hand, time spent with patients decreases with increased size, perhaps because there are more individual administrators and levels of bureaucracy to absorb malcontents.

Just as there are unique profiles associated with particular sizes, there are some notable consistencies across all categories. For example, the time spent on extramural activities varies only slightly with size. The same is true of meetings with representatives of professional organizations and staff unions, and discussions with superiors. Dealing with subordinates, although it takes up more of the time of administrators in 100-199 bed facilities, stands out as the major consumer of administrative attention regardless of the facility size. Except for the percent of time spend dealing with patients, there is little difference in the profiles of administrators of the smallest and the largest institutions.[10]

## Three Types of Facilities

The preceding discussion of the effect of size of work activity suggests there is some variation from small to large facilities. However, size of facility is not independent; that is, there are other conditions which vary closely with numbers of beds. As Table 16 reveals, there is a very strong association between size and type of ownership. Privately owned, for-profit facilities tend to be small (under 100 beds), while facilities operated by local, state and federal agencies (such as the Veterans Administration) are large (700 and more beds). The nonprofit so-called "community" or "volunteer" facilities are represented in all but the largest category of size.

The proprietary category contains all of the convalescent hospitals (16 facilities from which 17 interviews were obtained) as well as three acute general care hospitals and one industrial out-patient clinic.[11] (For sample composition by type of facility, see Table 1.)

The nonprofit category combines 35 respondents from 10 different facilities with 14 administrators from three different health maintenance organization facilities. Five administrators of as many specialized out-patient clinics complete the 54 total respondents in this category.

Table 16

Composition of Sample by Size and Type of Facility

| Number of Beds | Proprietary | Nonprofit | Government | Total Sample |
|---|---|---|---|---|
| None | 4.5 | 13.0 | 0 | 7.2 |
| 1-99 | 63.7 | 1.9 | 0 | 13.5 |
| 100-199 | 27.3 | 24.1 | 0 | 17.1 |
| 200-399 | 4.5 | 46.2 | 2.9 | 24.3 |
| 400-699 | 0 | 14.8 | 34.3 | 18.0 |
| 700 or more | 0 | 0 | 62.8 | 19.9 |
| Total Number of Cases | 22 | 54 | 35 | 111 |

The gross distinction between "private" (proprietary) and "public" (nonprofit) ownership apparently is associated with differences in administrative behavior, in part stemming from aggregate differences in patient services and size also associated with private/public status. Heydebrand notes that "public hospitals, in contrast to private ones, are larger, have a somewhat longer average length of stay, and lower personnel/patient and nurse/patient ratios."[12] Ruchlin, Pointer and Cannedy report some differences in administering profit and nonprofit institutions, but conclude that there are many administrative similarities.[13]

The seven facilities which comprise the government category include the largest institutions of the sample. But we must not draw the inference that the respondent profiles of the administrators from such facilities are a function of the effects of size alone. As we noted above (note 9), in certain types of government facilities such as mental and TB hospitals, increased size is not associated with organizational specialization and division of labor, conditions that make for communications and personnel management problems.

There are peculiar constraints on decision making in addition to size which play on the administrators of government institutions. For reasons we shall explore below, government hospitals have relatively low de jure and de facto operational autonomy; that is, they rank low in terms of both resources and ability to make independent decisions about resource allocations.[14]

Within the government category, there is a significant difference between the short term general care and extended care specialized institutions. The former tend to be much more similar in operational characteristics (if not in clientele and external resource providers) to nonprofit facilities of comparable size. But governmental extended care institutions have distinctive problems. In the present sample, two types of government extended care facilities are found: Veterans Administration and state mental. VA facilities are staffed with Civil Service personnel and medical personnel appointed by the Department of Medicine and Surgery; departmental specialization is highest in VA hospitals of any general category of institution; each hospital is linked into a larger federal agency through a complex hierarchy that exercises powerful (external) control over institutional resources; and VA hospitals have a special patient population that requires a more comprehensive "total institutional" form of care than is provided by other types of institutions.[15]

State mental facilities, which share the specialized patient requirements and provide many of the same services as VA hospitals, nevertheless have unique operational constraints. Perrow says that "the large, public mental hospital is a remarkably inefficient organization, as has been demonstrated repeatedly."[16] This stems from both internal and external circumstances:

> The state mental hospital is a resource-deprived institution, more or less treated as a necessary evil by those responsible for its support. The surrounding community and the communities it

serves are generally ignorant of its problems, needs, and practices. The superintendent of the state hospital is usually a doctor, often a psychiatrist. Below him fan out two largely incompatible hierarchies, the business-administrative and the medical-treatment. The business side often runs the hospital by virtue of its control over scarce resources, namely those required for the physical maintenance of the institution.[17]

That mental facility administrators operate in resource structures basically dissimilar to that of their colleagues in general hospitals has been illustrated by others.[18]

While one-third of the respondents in the government category is drawn from VA and mental facilities, the remainder is distributed throughout facilities of varying size. Moreover, the nonprofit group counts within it individuals in the main drawn from middle-sized HMO's and community hospitals. Thus we see that comparison by type of facility is not independent of size.

## Demographic Variations

Before examining the activity profiles of the administrators from propietary, nonprofit, and government facilities, we must ascertain whether or not there are major demographic variations in the groups that might bias the profiles. In the nonprofit and government groups the occupational categories are fairly evenly distributed; however, the proprietary group contains all of the convalescent administrators. Since we have previously established that this occupational group has a particular activity profile, attribution of variation in the present analysis to type of facility would be spurious. Determining whether convalescent administration per se or proprietary ownership is the controlling variable (or, indeed, some other variable or variables we have not isolated) awaits the comparison of proprietary and nonproprietary convalescent administrators, a task we are unable to perform.

We have already seen (Table 2) that over half of the

women of the sample (55.6%) are found in nonprofit facilities. However, when we ask what proportion of each group is female, we find no significant difference: 27.3% of the proprietary, 27.8% of the nonprofit, and 17.1% of the government administrators. Thus there is little bias introduced by sex variations among the samples.

Similarly, there is no significant variation among the three categories according to median length of tenure in their present positions (i.e., job turnover rate), percent reporting previous health administration experience, age, or level of professional identification.

Save for a slightly lower percent of college degrees among proprietary administrators, there is little variation in level of educational attainment. However, there is an interesting variation in post-graduate education. As Table 17 shows, government administrators report not only the highest percent of post-graduate education but also the highest percent of public administration specializations. While nonprofit facility administrators aggregate the highest percent of hospital

Table 17

Post Graduate College Major or Degree by Type of Facility

| Degree or Major | Proprietary | Nonprofit | Government | Total Sample |
|---|---|---|---|---|
| None | 59.1 | 38.9 | 28.6 | 39.6 |
| Business Adm | 4.5 | 3.7 | 5.7 | 4.5 |
| Hospital Adm | 4.5 | 20.4 | 8.6 | 13.5 |
| Public Adm | 0 | 5.6 | 22.9 | 10.0 |
| Other | 31.9 | 31.4 | 34.2 | 32.4 |
| Total Number of Cases | 22 | 54 | 35 | 111 |

administration majors, proprietary administrators break the symmetry of the pattern by ignoring business administration.

With the exception of the variations introduced by the appearance of all convalescent administrators in the "proprietary" category, there are no significant demographic differences in the composition of the groups from the three types of facilities. Thus what differences there may be among the three categories probably are not accountable to a disproportionate appearance in one group of one or more characteristics such as females, youth, high professional identification, or long tenure personnel. (We should bear in mind, however, that facility type is rather closely associated with size. Since size is closely related to function and not to personnel variables, size may be seen as part of the overall influence of the institution upon the administrative cadre—the impact of which we are attempting to evaluate.)

With these caveats about the composition of the three categories of facilities in mind, we shall now turn to an analysis of the relationship between type of facility and work activities.

## Facility Type and Administrative Activities

Because of the almost complete overlap of the present "proprietary" with the "convalescent hospital administrator" categories, we will not expand appreciably on the preceding discussion of the particular situational constraints, role partners, and work routines of this group of administrators. We shall, however, point out major variations among proprietary, nonprofit, and government profiles.

Table 18 demonstrates that there is little or no difference in the percent of time spent on selected activities among administrators of nonprofit and government facilities. As we noted above, convalescent hospital administrators, here presented as "proprietary" facility administrators, spend more time with patients and less time reading or preparing reports

Table 18

Percent of Average Day Allocated to Selected Activities

By Type of Facility

| Activity | Proprietary | Nonprofit | Government | Total Sample |
|---|---|---|---|---|
| Discussing Work Situation With Subordinates | 20.0 | 23.3 | 21.2 | 22.6 |
| Preparing Reports | 6.6 | 12.4 | 11.5 | 11.1 |
| Attending Staff Meetings | 5.4 | 10.4 | 12.6 | 10.2 |
| Correspondence and Telephone | 10.4 | 8.7 | 11.7 | 10.1 |
| Extramural Activities | 6.0 | 7.3 | 9.1 | 7.7 |
| Reading Reports | 4.0 | 7.4 | 9.8 | 7.6 |
| Discussing Unit's Activities with Superior | 7.9 | 7.5 | 6.9 | 7.5 |
| Dealing with Patients and/or Their Family | 20.5 | 4.3 | 2.8 | 7.1 |
| Meeting Representatives of Professional Associations and Staff Organizations and Unions | 8.6 | 4.9 | 7.0 | 6.4 |
| Total Number of Cases | 22 | 54 | 35 | 111 |

and attending staff meetings. But even the proprietary profile is not strikingly dissimilar from the other two.

Administrators in government facilities apparently spend the least amount of time dealing with patients or their families. This seems to contradict the speculation that the extended care facility provides more services to patients and, therefore, is more likely to be involved in patient-related difficulties that generate contact with administrators. I suspect that this *is* in fact the case; the smaller median percent of time reported for government administrators reflects the greater specialization of function that is associated with greater size: proportionately more of the government category department heads and administrative assistants are community relations, security, and other "staff" personnel whose responsibilities and duties involve few contacts with patients. Fewer of such "staff" administrators (and more "line" or patient-related administrators) are found in the smaller facilities from which the nonprofit category derives.

Government administrators spend somewhat more time dealing with extramural activities, attending staff meetings, reading reports, handling correspondence and telephoning, and meeting representatives of professional associations and staff unions—that is, *communicating*. With respect to the last two activities, the nonprofit administrator's profile stands apart from that of both the government and proprietary respondent's. On the other hand, nonprofit and government profiles report more time in staff meetings, preparing reports, and reading reports, but less time dealing with patients than do proprietary administrators. The latter category is composed largely of small-sized convalescent facilities, a condition we believe to be accountable for its different profile for reasons discussed above.

While there is little significant difference in the way administrators of nonprofit and government facilities spend their time, there is considerable variation in the problems they deal with and the role partners with which they interact. We shall explore these patterns in the following chapters.

The activity profile of the overall sample reveals that health administrators spend the greatest part of their working day (22.6%) discussing the work situation with their subordinates. One-third of their day is consumed by preparing reports, attending staff meetings, and telephoning and handling correspondence. The remainder is devoted to reading reports, discussing responsibilities with superiors, dealing with patients or families, and attending to extramural activities (about 7% for each of these).

While the percent of time spent in each of the above activities is similar for all four occupational categories, we noticed a distinctive profile for convalescent hospital administrators. They spend five or six times more of their work day dealing with patients or the family of patients than the other groups. However, they only spend one-third as much as DAs, CAOs, and AAs attending staff meetings and reading reports. These differences for convalescent administrators seems attributable to the limited subordinate staffs and the absence of medical practices and clinical procedures in their facilities.

Activities vary not only according to occupation but also by size of the facility. Administrators of large facilities spend more time preparing and reading reports and attending staff meetings than do their colleagues in smaller facilities. Time spent with patients decreases with increased size. This indicates that greater bureaucratization is associated with greater size; that is, there are more functionally specific jobs and services requiring more offices charged with supervision and control in larger facilities.

The type of facility in which the administrator works seems to be related to the types of activities that fill his day. The administrator of local, state, and federal institutions spends less time dealing with patients and more time attending to extramural activities, telephoning and handling correspondence, and meeting representatives of professional associations and staff unions than his counterparts in the other facility types. (This latter duty, as we shall see below, stems from the greater prevalence of labor unions and associations in government facilities.) The administrator of non-profit facilities spends less time handling communications and dealing with labor representatives, but otherwise his profile is similar to that of the government administrator's. Both are substantially different from the profile of the proprietary administrator.

While most of the proprietary administrators of the present sample are drawn from convalescent hospitals, it seems that the distinctive profile of the category would be largely unchanged if we were to draw another sample exclusively from acute care, short term proprietary hospitals. This is because the proprietary sector of the acute care industry is characterized by several distinctive structural features: namely, a mean bed size of about 38% and 53% for voluntary nonprofit and state and local government hospitals, respectively. Moreover, proprietary hospitals have only 85% of the other facilities average ratio of full-time personnel per 100 patients. Thus it seems reasonable to suggest that the administrators of these smaller facilities have fewer subordinate personnel to deal with, as well as fewer complicated medical procedures and laboratory processes to administer. (The absence of sophisticated equipment and the human support they require, and the absence of a good many administrative offices and problems is further suggested by the fact that the average financial assets per bed of proprietary hospitals are one half or less than that of the other two types of facilities.)

If this line of reasoning is valid, we would expect the hypothetical sample of proprietary administrators to report less time in staff management functions and more time with patient-related problems. The profiles of the government and nonprofit administrators reflect the wider range of medical, clinical, and administrative services their larger, richer facilities provide.

# NOTES

1. R. Schultz and A. C. Johnson, "Conflict in Hospitals," *Hospital Administration* 16 (1971), 38.

2. A. F. Wessen, "Hospital Ideology and Communication Between Ward Personnel," in E. G. Jaco (ed.) *Patients, Physicians and Illness,* 2nd. ed. (New York: Free Press, 1972), 325-342.

3. D. S. Pomrinse, "To What Degree are Hospitals Publically Accountable?" *Hospitals* 43 (1969), 41-44.

4. M. I. Roemer, "Education for Medical Care Administration," *Hospital Administration* 10 (1965), 11.

5. On the evolving nature of the convalescent hospital administrator's role, see R. L. Able, "Current Status of the Profession of Nursing Home Administration," *Journal of the American College of Nursing Home Administrators* 1 (1973), 3-10.

6. J. T. Gentry, et al., "Perceptual Differences of Administrators

Regarding the Importance of Health Programs: Implications for Education for Health Services Administration," *American Journal of Public Health* 60 (1970), 1006-1017.

7. T. R. Anderson and Seymour Warkov, "Organizational Size and Functional Complexity: A Study of Administration in Hospitals," *American Sociological Review* 26 (1961), 23-28.

8. W. V. Heydebrand, *Hospital Bureaucracy: A Comparative Study of Organizations* (New York: Dunellen, 1973), 237-253 and passim.

9. Heydebrand provides an elaborate analysis of the concomitants of size and offers exceptions to this general hypothesis. Speaking of psychiatric and other extended care facilities, "even though they may be large and have many subunits, such subunits tend to be structurally similar so that growth in size leads to an increase in structural and compositional homogeneity. In these hospitals therefore, the relative size of the administrative-clerical staff remains small and tends to decrease with growing size, with the exception of the very large size categories, where a slight increase in administrative specialization can be observed" (Hydebrand, *Hospital Bureaucracy,* 252).

10. An interesting theoretical treatment of the size/function/organizational structure issue is offered by B. H. Mayhew and W. A. Rushing, "Occupational Structure of Community General Hospitals: The Harmonic Series Model," *Social Forces* 51 (1973), 455-461.

11. The proprietary segment of the industry, especially in the convalescent hospital sector, has grown in recent years. Kovner reports that "since 1968, business corporations have entered the hospital industry, and the proprietary share of facilities may increase. Thirty-eight companies now control more than 25 percent of the proprietary hospitals and nearly 40 percent of the proprietary beds. These corporations now own 19,000 beds and have planned, as of 1970, to add or construct an additional 14,000 beds." A. R. Kovner, "The Hospital Administrator and Organizational Effectiveness," in B. S. Georgopoulos (ed.) *Organization Research on Health Institutions* (Ann Arbor: University of Michigan, Institute for Social Research, 1972), 356. On the expansion of proprietary convalescent hospitals, see P. W. Earle, "The Nursing Home Industry," *Hospitals* 44 (1970), 45-51, 60-66. An article in the *Wall Street Journal,* 27 November 1972, suggests that invester interest in proprietary corporations may be cooling. See D. Dorfman, "Heard on the Street."

Among acute care, short term facilities, the percent of proprietary hospitals has steadily declined since 1946 until it now accounts for approximately ten percent of the nation's facilities. And the actual number of such facilities has actually declined steadily. For a discussion of the proprietary side of the industry, see B. Steinwald and D.

Neuhauser, "The Role of the Proprietary Hospital," *Law and Contemporary Problems* 35 (1970), 817-838. (Current figures on the number of proprietary hospitals may be found in the annual "Guide Issue" of *Hospitals,* the organ of the American Hospital Association.)

12. Heydebrand, *Hospital Bureaucracy,* 144.

13. H. S. Ruchlin, D. D. Pointer, and L. L. Cannedy, "Administering Profit and Nonprofit Institutions," *Hospital Progress* 54 (1973), 80.

14. Heydebrand, *Hosital Bureaucracy,* 287-288.

15. Ibid., 115, 181, 243, 243-246.

16. C. Perrow, "Hospitals: Technology, Structure, and Goals," in J. March (ed.) *Handbook of Organizations* (Chicago: Rand McNally, 1965), 926.

17. Perrow, "Hospitals," 921. The dual occupational identity of the psychiatrist-administrator, like that of the physician-administrator, subjects him to intense contradictory role-expectations—one set from his medical staff, another from his administrative subordinates. See I. Belknap, *Human Problems of a State Mental Hospital* (New York: McGraw-Hill, 1956): "The superintendent is continually torn between his obligations as a professional man and as an institutional executive" (p. 242, note 4).

18. Cf., H. Ah and S. Mailick, "Training for Mental Health Administrators," *Hospital and Community Psychiatry* 22 (1971), 348-352; I. Belknap and J. Steinle, *The Community and Its Hospitals* (Syracuse: Syracuse University Press, 1963); W. Caudill, *The Psychiatric Hospital as a Small Society* (Cambridge: Harvard University Press, 1958); Amitai Etzioni, "Authority Structure and Organizational Effectiveness," *Administrative Science Quarterly* 4 (1959), 43-67; Ibid., "Interpersonal and Structural Factors in the Study of Mental Hospitals," *Psychiatry* 23 (1960), 13-22; S. Feldman (ed.) *The Administration of Mental Health Services* (Springfield, Ill.: Charles C. Thomas, 1973); R. W. Hawkes, "The Role of the Psychiatric Administrator," *Administrative Science Quarterly* 6 (1961), 89-107; J. Henry, "The Formal Structure of a Psychiatric Hospital," *Psychiatry* 17 (1954), 139-151; A. H. Stanton and M. F. Schwartz, *The Mental Hospital* (New York: Basic Books, 1954).

*Chapter 5*

# MAJOR PROBLEMS

Reviewing how health administators spend their time, we discovered that they are largely occupied with activities of essentially a communications nature—discussion with subordinates and superiors, attending meetings, handling correspondence and reports. In this chapter we shall probe the contents and causes of communications: What are the typical problems health care administrators deal with? Are these problems found throughout the profession? What are the origins of these major time-consuming interactions?

Two separate measures were employed to seek the roots of the administrators' activities. One was an open-ended question which sought the respondents' perceptions of their environment: "What are the major problems that you have to deal with in this job? That is, the main task you have to handle?" The respondents were encouraged to reflect upon their responsibilities and assignments and to produce their answers in their own terms and at as much length as they desired. The largely verbatim responses of all respondents were subjected to a content analysis to determine the major common problems they contained. These profiles were then categorized so as to reveal not only the type of problem (for example, "budgeting" or "inadequate information upon which to base my decisions") but also the role partners involved (for example, "medical staff" or "subordinates").

The second method of determining the content and source of administrators' problems was a series of directed questions: "Now I'm going to mention some problems or issues that some administrators have said they have. I would like you to tell me whether or not they are problems for you. In other words, do you have to handle any of these matters in your present job?" Then each respondent was asked, "Is determining costs of patient services and care a major problem?" "Do patients ever cause you any problems?" and other questions about specific role partners. The series of questions covered both the major responsibilities of administration (budgeting, personnel management, industrial relations, etc.), as well as the major sectors or holders of resources which form structural partnerships with health administrators (physicians, nurses, boards of trustees, associations and organizations).

The two questioning techniques produced a wide range of items. In order to reduce the list to a comprehensible proportion, only problems mentioned or affirmed by 10% or more of the overall sample are dealt with here. The same cutoff shall be employed with the identification of sectors. Before reviewing the results of the research, let us note some items which did not survive the cutoff.

## Infrequently Cited Problems

The obligations of the health industry to play a progressive role in the local and national community, to be sensitive to community needs and preferences, and to work creatively with representatives of the community are increasingly performed by health care administrators. The three or four largest institutions in the present study have assigned administrators part- or full-time responsibility for community relations. Overall, few health care administrators mentioned problems with their facility's community or in reconcilling their administrative duties with what we previously referred to as their civic responsibilities. Moreover, dealing directly with the local social, economic, and political elites, or local government officials is restricted to a very small element of CAOs of the larger nonprofit and government facilities.

State and federal government agencies that regulate health care facilities or that allocate funds for health programs are dealt with by a tiny fraction of administrators. Here again only a few chief administrative officers, or individuals assigned particular programmatic responsibilities (such as negotiating a building grant or handling Medicare or Medicaid reimbursement) reported problems with government representatives.

Similarly, interactions with third party payers, representatives of equipment and service vendors, and representatives of private foundations—three sectors that are possible sources of funds, information, new technology, prestige and other resources—are restricted and not reported by the overall sample.

Now we shall turn to the major problems which emerged from the overall sample. We shall structure the analysis around functional topics and compare the profiles of the sample's occupational, size, and type of facility categories.

### Bugeting and Finance

In response to the open-ended question, "What major problems do you have to deal with?", nearly one-half of the respondents volunteered some aspect of bookkeeping, accounting, fiscal management, budgeting or financial difficulties. In terms of frequency of mention, budgeting and finance far surpass (48.6%) the second most frequently mentioned problem, regulations or laws (23.4%).

There are several aspects of the budget and finance problem. One is the difficulty that arises from simply having to keep track of appropriations: seeing who spends how much of what fund on which accounts. For individuals lacking accounting or other finance management skills, bookkeeping or budgeting can be an unintelligible enigma. Another problem is the necessity of weighing requests for allocations from competing programs or individuals. Here the health care administrator is in a position not unlike that of the congress person serving on the Armed Services Appropriations Committee: specialists, armed with imposing figures, clothed in technical expertise, and practiced in manipulating virtue, justice and credibility, appear and demand support, in the name of Ultimate Survival, for *their* particular proposals. Like the congress person, the health care administrator has limited resources and an over-supply of demands; he must run the risk of funding boondoggles while starving worthwhile projects; and he must make judgments although he lacks basic information or technical knowledge of the proffered alternatives.

Aside from the inherent difficulties in preparing budgets and keeping track of expenditures, health care administrators bear extra burdens imposed by third party payers. The federal government, one prominent "third party payer" (e.g., Medicare), demands strict cost-accounting procedures as a condition of payment. For example, "principle 2-3 of the Medicare formula states that providers receiving payment on the basis of 'reasonable costs' must provide adequate cost data. These must be related to financial and statistical records capable of verification by qualified auditors and based on an approved method of cost finding."[1]

Another dimension of budget and finance problems derives from the administrator's inability to exercise cost/benefit control over the institution's services. Kovner's observations illustrate the predicament of the administrator, responsible for resource allocations but deprived of effective authority:

> Many decisions regarding costs and the financing of operations, such as the level of reimbursement for care of indigent patients and for educational expenses, are not controllable by the administrator.
>
> Other decisions are controllable at the hospital level, but the administrator generally lacks the authority to make them. It has been estimated that 10% to 20% of the patients in the hospital on any one day do not need to be there. Despite utilization committees and additional extended care facilities, this is probably so in 1970 [and 1974 as well]. The hospital administrator cannot directly influence physicians to perform fewer procedures and order fewer tests, or readily induce insured patients to utilize doctors' and hospital services less.[2]

Kovner's speculation about the inability of the administrator to control costs is supported by the responses to two directed questions. When asked if they had services which operated at a loss, and if determining patients' charges or costs was a problem, an affirmative reply was obtained from 70% and 90% of the sample respectively.

## Regulations and Laws

Problems associated with regulations and laws were mentioned by almost one-quarter of the sample. Doubtless, many had in mind the complex reimbursement, eligibility, and record-keeping requirements set down in Medicare legislation. (Close to 60% of the sample affirmed that Medicare caused them "special problems.")

But Medicare is only the tip of the iceberg. Regulations are imposed by both governmental agencies, and licensing and accreditation bodies. Somers reports that

> a recent listing by an official of the American Hospital Association identified sixty-eight different hospital programs or facilities affected by direct government control. . . .

The AHA study listed sixteen different federal agencies involved in hospital regulation of one sort or another, nine state government bodies typically involved, and twelve local government bodies. In addition, many nongovernmental bodies, such as the Joint Commission on Accreditation of Hospitals and the numerous specialized accrediting bodies—the American Medical Association, the Association of American Medical Colleges, the National League for Nursing, etc.—exercise what amounts to compulsory standard-setting for the better hospitals.[3]

While we tend to think of rules and laws that affect the operations of health care facilities as the product of regulatory and legislative action, there is another body of law which is becoming increasingly important to health care administrators. This is the tort law which is formed through judicial verdicts and which establishes the extent and type of liability to which the health institution is subject. Recent judicial decisions have made possible action against the facility per se, not just the physician. Hospitals themselves are subject to six and seven figure judgments arising from negligence.

But to further complicate the life of the health care administrator, "not only have the courts begun to breach the distinction between provision of facilities and care, but they have begun to insist that hospitals have a duty to enforce *proper* medical standards, not just local community practices."[4] *Quality,* in other words, may be a judicable criterion. The administrator shares with the medical staff the responsibility, but probably shoulders more of the burden, for seeing to it that the facility avoids liability and culpability for deficient or substandard performance.[5]

Other areas of health care administration that fall under public authority include the investment of endowments, the tax-exempt status of certain types of corporations, management of employee retirement funds, and the staffing of the facility in accordance with fair employment practice requirements. This latter point, related as it is to the necessity of demonstrable proof that racial or sexual discrimination is not being practiced, has emerged in the 1970s as potentially a very troublesome issue. This is partly because many health care facilities (especially "community" hospitals, nonprofit, and government) are located in areas of high ethnic minority concentration. As a result of traditional occupational and educational bias, many health care facilities find their unskilled work forces largely or exclusively non-Anglo, while their technical and professional occupations become whiter as the salary increases.[6] Hospitals and other health delivery facilities can look forward to increasing pressure, both from local communities and public agencies, to implement successful affirmative action programs.

## Information

Given the volume of reports required, the hours spent in verbal and written communication, and the specialized, often highly technical nature of many assignments, it should not come as a surprise that 15.3% of the sample volunteered that absence of data or inadequate communications was a problem for them. When asked if they obtained information when they needed it to complete their assignment (i.e., at the "right time"), 26.1% replied negatively.

Even these figures, in the absence of data or information, disguise the profound impact that the mismanagement of communications has on the administrator. At the core of administration is the necessity to make decisions, that is, to choose from among alternative courses of action. Without accurate, timely information, no decisionmaker, regardless of his intellectual and professional accomplishments, can act to generate effective, efficient exchanges of resources. How much of the problem with budgeting and finance management has its roots in inaccurate or unavailable data? How many of the problems with rules and laws originate in the inability of key personnel to receive communications or to obtain intelligible information? And how many of the difficulties and misunderstandings with employees arise from their missing instructions, or from communications which were not clearly understood? Many of the problems involving patients are derived from the inability of the complex bureaucratic organization, which creates vast amounts of information, to deliver Mrs. Smith's salt-free breakfast or to find Mr. Brown's medical records. And as technology continues to produce ever-more sophisticated curative and administrative procedures, equipment and support systems, the vulnerability of the administrator to misplaced or distorted data and communications increases—perhaps at an exponential rate.

Modern technology, with its promise of better health care and improved health care administration, looms as more of a threat than a saviour—or at least this seems to be the case judging from the problems administrators report with current technology.

## Technology

In allocating funds, top level health care administrators must grapple with the relative advantages of purchasing, leasing, or doing without a whole range of advanced medical technologies and the 5,000 medical devices available: hyperbaric chambers, defibrillators, cobalt units, scintillation counters, and the like. All administrators are faced with the task of integrating new technologies and devices into work units, reviewing their contributions to the unit's activities, and deciding what items and procedures should be improved. In the nonclinical, nontechnical units of health care facilities, administrators are faced with computer technology management science advances that have far-reaching implications for health service delivery, planning, and evaluation.[7] The ubiquitous computer is now used in patient billing,[8] clinic scheduling,[9] personnel management,[10] medical records shortage and retrieval,[11] systems operations research,[12] facility planning, [13] food service planning, [14] and cost/benefit analysis. [15]

Aside from new procedures, technical advances spawn the redefinition of relations between administrators and other actors within the health care institution. For example, closed circuit television, patient monitoring systems, and two-way communication systems have greatly increased the centralization of nursing stations vis-a-vis the administrative hierarchy. In the past the individual nurse moved around the ward, talking with other staff members and relying on interactions with them to perform her duties; now many nurses remain largely stationary, relying on technology rather than personal interaction for information and for carrying out many of their tasks. Technology allows the nurses to marshall many resources under their immediate control, thereby making them less dependent on, and less easily controlled by, administrators (and other co-workers). [16]

Individual respondents touched on some of these problems when they complained about not understanding computer capabilities, having difficulties with physicians or department heads who wished to purchase new equipment or refused to use available systems, and finding it difficult to recruit and retain skilled technicians and laboratory specialists. But the real magnitude of the technology problem appeared in the responses to the question: "Does the rapidly changing and growing sophistication of medical equipment and technology cause you any particular problems?" Over 57% of the sample replied "yes."

It would be useful to explore just how much of the time spent with subordinates or what percent of the problems with the medical staff, finance, personnel management and the other major problems cited by respondents have their roots in the administrator's inability to comprehend and manage medical technology and related programs. Such a study would help to clarify much of the uncertainty involved in educating health care administrators. There is little if any exposure to medical technology—especially the more ad-

vanced forms of it—in the contemporary health care administration curriculum. And few in the present sample have had
much experience on the job. Presently only the largest and
most complex institutions use third generation computers
and the latest medical and clinical hardware. Most of the
present sample is not drawn from these vanguard institutions.
So our sample has not been exposed to much that is in store
for them. What will be the impact on the administrator when
advanced technologies are extended to the smaller general
hospitals and convalescent hospitals? And what steps should
be taken to prepare the next generation of health care
administrators?

## Problems By Occupational Category

As Table 19 indicates, the problems which stand out in the
mind of the administrator vary according to his position or
occupation. Among the four major categories, convalescent
hospital administrators have the most distinctive profile. Inadequate data, facility planning and supervision, and technology are much less frequently mentioned or affirmed as
problems. Medicare and regulations and laws, however, are
cited as problems well above the rate among the overall
sample. These convalescent facilities, which are smaller and
provide few clinical and technological services, have recently
become the subject of much new legislation and regulatory
activity by local, state, and federal agencies; and because
most, if not all, of their patients are old enough to be
potential Medicare beneficiaries, they more often have problems with eligibility, repayment, records, and so forth. In
addition, licensing of both the administrator and the facility
creates new and perplexing difficulties for many convalescent
administrators.[17]

Chief administrative officers less frequently complain
about poor data or communications; perhaps they put pressure on their subordinates to produce the needed materials

Table 19

Problems by Occupational Category

| Problem | Convalescent Hospital Adm | Chief Adm Short Term & Extended Care Hospitals | Department Adm | Administrative Assistant | Outpatient Clinic Adm | Total Sample |
|---|---|---|---|---|---|---|
| "What major problems do you have to deal with...?" | (Percent mentioning) | | | | | |
| Budgeting & Finance | 41.2 | 45.5 | 55.8 | 47.8 | 33.3 | 48.6 |
| Regulations & Laws | 35.3 | 31.8 | 23.3 | 13.0 | 0 | 23.4 |
| Inadequate Data or Communications | 5.9 | 4.5 | 20.9 | 17.4 | 33.3 | 15.3 |
| Planning or Supervising Physical Plant | 5.9 | 22.7 | 7.0 | 17.4 | 0 | 11.7 |
| "Do you have a problem with...?" | (Percent Affirming) | | | | | |
| Services Operating at a Loss | 64.7 | 86.4 | 60.5 | 87.0 | 33.3 | 70.3 |
| Medicare | 88.2 | 72.7 | 55.8 | 34.8 | 50.0 | 59.5 |
| Medical Equipment or Technology | 5.9 | 68.2 | 62.8 | 87.0 | 16.7 | 57.7 |
| Determining Patient Charges or Costs | 58.8 | 45.5 | 32.6 | 39.1 | 16.7 | 39.6 |
| Obtaining Information at the Right Time | 17.6 | 22.7 | 27.9 | 30.4 | 33.3 | 26.1 |
| Total Number of Cases | 17 | 22 | 43 | 23 | 6 | 111 |

and receive better information. CAOs tend to spend their time with complex, novel, or "crisis" problems—ones that involve such a range of actors, magnitude of resources, or number of dimensions that only the most senior executive authority can deal with them. Accordingly, ascertaining eligibility, negotiating with the Social Security Administration, and bargaining with review committees over Medicare patients is a very frequent problem for CAOs. Likewise, they are much more frequently involved in facility expansion and utilization problems because the former involves great outlays of capital, and the latter involves the medical staff as well as other resources.

It is instructive to compare the profiles of CAOs and AAs because both categories are essentially administrative generalists. The data suggest that the latter may well screen mundane problems from the former. On the other hand, the more senior executives apparently take jurisdiction in some matters, removing them from their junior colleagues' responsibilities. For example, communications problems involving several departments and technology problems requiring major expenditures are taken care of by the CAOs; matters of regulation and Medicare by the AAs.

The department heads, because of the relatively narrow, often specialized tasks their units perform, are less prone to mention problems with such integrative, facility-wide responsibilities as facility planning or supervision, the profitability of specific services, or determination of service costs and patient charges. DAs cite problems stemming from Medicare much less often than do the CAO group. Department heads, however, more frequently volunteer information regarding difficulties with budgeting and finance matters. The difference here is not large and it may reflect a medical version of the "Peter Principle."[18] Professor Peter has observed that people are often promoted past their level of competence. Because an individual is a superior technician, nurse, or cook, he or she is made supervisor of the unit. However the skills and experiences which permitted him or her to excel as a worker are of little direct or immediate use in the new position. In looking at the career patterns of department heads, we find that several have come to their present job with no previous administrative experience. It is true that a slightly larger percent of administrative assistants likewise report no previous administrative experience; however, the inexperienced AAs were on their first job. The department heads without previous experience were recruited from clinical, technical, or clerical jobs. The point is that some fraction of department heads have found themselves in positions requiring them to plan and execute budgets, to file financial reports and to keep records, but they lack preparation for these administrative tasks.

To argue that these department administrators lack suitable preparation for successfully accomplishing administrative tasks is not to argue for staffing such positions with only administratively trained individuals. Such individuals would be in the opposite but equally debilitating bind: they would have little or no substantial information about the work of the unit, would be ill-equipped to discuss work problems with their subordinates, and would lack knowledge of the criteria of technical competence against which to evaluate their subordinates' performance. Obviously, an optimal blend is highly trained and seasoned individuals familiar with the department's responsibilities who have been introduced to and have had an opportunity to become familiar with the relevant administrative tools. Progressive institutions, seeing the need for such instruction, have developed in-service training for mid-career people seeking (or being sought for) middle and upper level administrative assignments. We shall return below to the issue of continuing training and educational preparation for health care administrators.

## Size and Type of Facility

Because of the association between size and type of facility (see Table 16), it is difficult to assess the independent effect of type of facility on problem profiles. Basing type on the ownership or authority structure of the facility (that is, whether control is invested in a proprietary corporation, a nonprofit corporation, or an agency of government) further complicates matters because the nature of patient services performed is not independent of type of control. To a large degree, the present study deals with proprietary facilities which are also convalescent hospitals, nonprofit hospitals which are also acute care, short-term general institutions, and government facilities which are either mental hospitals or Veterans Administration general hospitals with multiple extended care and special rehabilitory and other patient services.

Table 20

Problems by Size of Facility

| Problem | No Beds | 1 - 99 Beds | 100-199 Beds | 200-399 Beds | 400-699 Beds | 700 & more Beds | Total Sample |
|---|---|---|---|---|---|---|---|
| "What major problems do you have to deal with...?" | | | | (Percent Mentioning) | | | |
| Budgeting & Finance | 37.5 | 46.7 | 57.9 | 59.3 | 45.0 | 36.4 | 48.6 |
| Regulations & Laws | 12.5 | 20.0 | 15.8 | 29.6 | 20.0 | 31.8 | 23.4 |
| Inadequate Data or Communications | 50.0 | 13.3 | 10.5 | 7.4 | 15.0 | 22.7 | 15.3 |
| Planning or Supervising the Physical Plant | 12.5 | 13.3 | 5.3 | 14.8 | 15.0 | 9.1 | 11.7 |
| "Do you have a problem with...?" | | | | (Percent Affirming) | | | |
| Services Operating at a Loss | 50.0 | 73.3 | 42.1 | 88.9 | 85.0 | 54.5 | 70.3 |
| Medicare | 50.0 | 80.0 | 57.9 | 85.2 | 50.0 | 36.4 | 59.5 |
| Medical Equipment or Technology | 0 | 20.0 | 63.2 | 66.7 | 85.0 | 59.1 | 57.7 |
| Determing Patient Charges or Cost | 25.0 | 60.0 | 36.9 | 37.0 | 25.0 | 45.5 | 39.6 |
| Obtaining Information at the Right Time | 37.5 | 20.0 | 31.6 | 14.8 | 35.0 | 31.8 | 26.1 |
| Total Number of Cases | 8 | 15 | 19 | 27 | 20 | 22 | 111 |

Table 21

Problems by Type of Facility

| Problem | Proprietary | Nonprofit | Government | Total Sample |
|---|---|---|---|---|
| "What major problems do you have to deal with...?" | (Percent Mentioning) | | | |
| Budgeting and Finance | 50.0 | 53.7 | 40.0 | 48.6 |
| Regulations and Laws | 27.3 | 20.4 | 25.7 | 23.4 |
| Inadequate Data or Communications | 9.1 | 16.7 | 20.0 | 15.3 |
| Planning or Supervising Physical Plant | 9.1 | 13.0 | 11.4 | 11.7 |
| "Do you have a problem with...?" | (Percent Affirming) | | | |
| Services Operating at a Loss | 63.6 | 74.1 | 62.9 | 70.3 |
| Medicare | 81.8 | 64.8 | 42.9 | 59.5 |
| Medical Equipment or Technology | 22.7 | 61.1 | 71.4 | 57.7 |
| Determing Patient Charges or Costs | 59.1 | 29.6 | 40.0 | 39.6 |
| Obtaining Information at the Right time | 18.2 | 28.8 | 34.4 | 26.1 |
| Total Number of Cases | 22 | 54 | 35 | 111 |

The problem in interpreting Tables 20 and 21 comes from attempting to decide which is the controlling variable, size or type, or whether the two are independent. That is, do administrators of large short-term acute care facilities have essentially the same problems as administrators in similar sized Veterans Administration or government mental hospitals?

The present sample is too small to allow us to control simultaneously for the effects of size *and* type of facility. But perhaps we can gain a clue to the relative power of size and type (or service profile, which is closely related to type in the present case) from reviewing the findings of Heydebrand. His research of the relationships among size, occupational specialization, and departmental specialization is based on an analysis of data from 3,544 U.S. facilities. We shall summarize portions of it here.

Table 22 reveals that occupational specialization increases directly with increased size: the larger the facility, the more likely it is that it will offer a greater number of 39 specific occupational categories identified by Heydebrand. Increased occupational specialization, in turn, is related to greater ranges of technical and clinical as well as administrative services. Increased occupational specialization is associated with increased departmental specialization in the overall sample. The seven operational indicators of departmental specialization are the medical component (physicians), the professional nursing component, the subprofessional nursing component (practical nurses, aides, and attendants), the technical component (dietary, laundry, housekeeping, and maintenance personnel), and the administrative component (business and clerical personnel). Size correlates positively with increased departmental specialization in the overall sample, although at a lower level than does functional specialization.

Table 22

Intercorrelations Between Size, Occupational Specialization, and

Department Specialization in Teaching Hospitals

| | U.S. Hosp. | Total Sample | Voluntary General | Government Psychiatric | General | Veteran's Administration General |
|---|---|---|---|---|---|---|
| Size & Occupational Specialization | .75 | .74 | .82 | .67 | .83 | .54 |
| Size & Departmental Specialization | .29 | .30 | -.53 | -.79 | .52 | -.13 |
| Occupational Specialization & Departmental Specialization | .59 | .62 | .51 | -.44 | .61 | .14 |
| Total Number of Cases | 6,825 | 3,544 | 467 | 91 | 185 | 60 |

[1] Wolf V. Heydebrand, Hospital Bureaucracy: A Comparative Study of Organizations (New York: Dunellen, 1973), modification of Table 18, p. 172.

But when we look at the association between functional and departmental specialization and size, controlling for function (or in terms of the present study, *type*), we find a good deal of variation. Both measures of specialization correlate very positively with size among general service, short-term facilities. And among government psychiatric hospitals (as well as other categories of psychiatric institutions reported by Heydebrand but omitted from Table 22), occupational specialization increases with increased size. However, among psychiatric institutions size is *negatively* related to departmental specialization because the larger hospitals actually report fewer departments than smaller facilities.

Among Veterans Administration facilities, size is less strongly associated with occupational specialization and negatively associated with departmental specialization. It is important to remember that Veterans Administration facilities provide a much wider range of programs, including extended residence and rehabilitation services, than do general hospitals. VA facilities tend to combine the services provided independently by general and convalescent hospitals as well as specialized clinics, social welfare departments, and occupational and social rehabilitation centers. Because of their service profile, VA facilities manifest many of the characteristics of mental and psychiatric institutions.

Heydebrand concludes:

> A generalization which emerges from these findings is that unifunctional, specialized organizations (psychiatric institutions, specialized clinics, convalescent hospitals) tend to become structurally simpler as they increase in size, since the larger size usually implies a greater degree of internal homogeneity.
>
> By contrast, in organizations with multifunctional or diversified task structure (general hospitals, VA facilities), an increase in size is likely to entail not only an increase in functional specialization, but also in structural differentiation conducive to departmental specialization.[19]

In a multifunctional organization the ratio of administrative-supervisory personnel to other employees declines sharply with increased size. And this ratio also declines with increased occupational specialization, particularly in unifunctional organizations. At the same time, the importance of the overall coordinating function of professional administrators increases to the extent that hospitals change from doctor-centered institutions to multifunctional, diagnostic, and therapeutic service centers.[20]

In sum, what Heydebrand's analysis suggests is that size and type of facility are both independently related to particular administrative tasks because both are associated with occupational specialization. Occupational specialization points to more personnel and subspecializations, elaborate technological configurations, and a great array of services. These conditions are likely to be associated with greater integrating, coordinating, and resource allocating difficulties.

But type of facility (unifunctional or multifunctional) has an effect on administration independent of size. Neither departmentalization nor occupational specialization increases with size among psychiatric or VA facilities. This indicates that administrators in such facilities must deal with similar occupational groups, patient services, technology, and communications barriers arising from occupational status cleavage regardless of the number of beds they administer.

In light of this discussion, we can read Tables 20 and 21 as saying that little of the variation in the proprietary and government columns is attributable to the size of the facilities, but that much of the variation in the nonprofit column probably is. Conversely, the differences between the smallest and largest facility size columns would be substantially greater *if* we included only respondents from general care, short-term institutions regardless of whether their institutions were proprietary, nonprofit or governmental.

The present sample of health care administrators report few problems of a community-relations nature, few contacts with representatives of regulatory or government funding bodies, and few contacts with third party payers, vendors and suppliers, and private foundations. Nearly half the sample volunteered problems involving budgeting or finance. Over half of those interviewed cited special problems with Medicare; almost one-fourth mentioned problems arising from regulations or statutory restrictions. Because of the numerous and often detailed reports required of health care provider institutions, we speculated that some of the problems in meeting the requirements of law and regulatory bodies stem from the lack of information arriving from subordinates "at the right time." Over half of the sample responded affirmatively when asked if medical and administrative technology caused special problems. The implications of the technology revolution, especially the role of the computer in medicine and in management, have not been felt in many of the institutions from which our sample comes; thus, the real magnitude of the problems caused administrators by technology may not have been reflected in the present study.

There is some variation in response profiles by occupation; in particular, convalescent hospital administrators stand apart from their colleagues in other types of institutions. Between administrators of general and specialized hospitals (including HMOs), there is some variation in responses. We speculated that the difference might follow "staff" and "line" responsibilities, (although admittedly there is no clear separation). In particular, CAOs and AAs are charged with maintaining the overall institution; these two groups report a higher frequency of problems with plant maintenance and unprofitable services. The profile of the department administrator may well conceal variations between patient service and institutional maintenance units. Problems of personnel administrators or security department heads might be substantially different from those reported by the chief of nursing services, head dietician, or laboratory supervisor. There is some variation in activities between the two groups of administrative generalists: CAOs typically handle the more complex negotiations or novel programs while AAs deal with routine matters.[21]

Finally, we looked at the relation between size and type of

facility and problems mentioned. In order to help clarify the confusion caused by the strong association in the present study between size and function, we looked at research reported by Heydebrand. We concluded that both size and type of facility (that is, services provided which in the present study very closely follow type of ownership) are probably independently related to variations in problems because both are associated with variations in occupational and departmental specializations—that is, with problems of communications, integration, coordination, budgeting, and so forth which arise with more employees and greater division and specialization of services. At the same time, however, size and type of facility are interrelated insofar as they are associated with administrative problems, because in unifunctional institutions such as convalescent or mental hospitals, specialization does not necessarily increase, nor do problems of integration and coordination multiply, with increased size. (In fact, Heydebrand suggests that some types of administrative difficulties may actually decrease with increased size because units become more homogeneous as the institutions approach the upper limits of size.) Further research which controls for the effects of both size and function of the facility is needed to clarify the impact on administrators of the type and size of institutions.

# NOTES

1. A. R. Somers, *Hospital Regulation: The Dilemma of Public Policy* (Princeton: Princeton University, Industrial Relations Section, 1969), 171.

2. A. R. Kovner, "The Hospital Administrator and Organizational Effectiveness," in B. S. Georgopoulos (ed.) *Organization Research on Health Institutions* (Ann Arbor: University of Michigan, Institute for Social Research, 1972), 361-362.

3. Somers, *Hospital Regulation,* 16.

4. M. N. Zald and F. D. Hair, "The Social Control of General Hospitals," in B. S. Georgopoulos (ed.) *Organization Research on Health Institutions* (Ann Arbor: University of Michigan, Institute for Social Research, 1972), 63.

5. Of special concern to the administrator is the law as developed in the *Darling v. Charleston Community Memorial Hospital* (1965) case. Here the court extended liability to the hospital for failing to maintain a general (high) standard of care—even though the presumed standard of care which might be used to establish liability is higher than the georgraphic area's standard. What the court seems to have done was to charge hospital boards of directors (and, operationally, chief administrative officers) with the responsibility of overseeing that the facility lives up to a general standard, which may reasonably be inferred from the overall industry, in order to be free from joint and several liability in malpractice suits. See ibid., 63-66.

6. See W. V. D'Antonio and J. Samora, "Occupational Stratifications in Four Southwestern Communities: A Study of Ethnic Differential Employment in Hospitals," *Social Forces* 41 (1962), 18-24.

7. See P. F. Gross, "Development and Implementation of Health Care Technology: The U.S. Experience," *Inquiry* 9 (1972), 34-48.

8. J. Blanco, Jr., "Streamlined Billing for Medicare Outpatients," *Hospitals* 43 (1969), 50-52.

9. L. W. Cronkhite, Jr., "Computer Brings Order to Clinical Scheduling Systems," *Hospitals* 43 (1969), 55-56.

10. A. M. Powers and G. F. Whitelock, Jr., "Computerized Employee Data Aid Administrative Decision-Making," *Hospitals* 42 (1968), 60-63; C. L. Packer, "Automation in the Personnel Department," *Hospitals* 45 (1971), 45-48.

11. L. S. Davis, et al., "Computer-Stored Medical Records," *Computers and Biomedical Research* 1 (1968), 452-469; B. G. Lamson, et al., "Hospitalwide System for Handling Medical Data," *Hospitals* 41 (1967), 67-80.

12. R. Emrich and E. Zak, "Computer Assists in Utilization Reviews," *Hospitals* 42 (1968), 56-69; T. F. Keller, "The Hospital Information System," *Hospital Administration* 14 (1969), 40-50; D. Conley, "A Management Team Approach to Hospital Systems Analysis," *Hospital Administration* 15 (1970) 58-78.

13. J. R. Haggerty, "Computerized Information System: Acceleration of Hospital Planning," *Hospitals* 44 (1970), 43-46; J. J. Souder, "Computers Can Bring a New Rationality into Hospital Design," *Modern Hospital* 110 (1968), 80-86.

14. R. M. DeMarco, "Planning a Computer for a Food Service Department," *Hospitals* 42 (1968), 107-113; J. Andrews and H. B. Tuthill, "Computer-Based Management of Dietary Departments," *Hospitals* 42 (1968), 117-123; R. L. Gue, "Mathematical Basis for Computer Planned Non-Selective Menus," *Hospitals* 43 (1969), 102-104.

15. A. McCosh, "Computerized Cost Finding Systems," *Hospital Financial Management* 23 (1969), 18-22.

16. W. V. Heydebrand, *Hospital Bureaucracy: A Comparative Study of Organizations* (New York: Dunellen, 1973), 328.

17. See L. McCoy, "Licensing of Nursing Home Administrators," *Medical Care* 9 (1971), 127-135; W. W. Rogers, *General Administration in the Nursing Home* (Boston: Cahners, 1972); M. J. Stoots (ed.) *Education for Administration in Long Term Care Facilities* (Washington, D.C.: Association of University Programs in Hospital Administration, 1973), especially D. J. Perkins, "Education for the Licensed Professional Practice of Nursing Home Administration," 140-156.

18. See L. J. Peter and R. Hull, *The Peter Principle: Why Things Always Go Wrong* (New York: William Morrow, 1969).

19. Heydebrand, *Hospital Bureaucracy,* 178-179.

20. Ibid., 211.

21. It is likely that Associate Administrators and Administrative Assistants are seen by their co-workers in the hospital and by themselves as separate elements in the administrative cadre. Our research indicates that they perform services and deal with problems which combine to form a distinctive activities' profile. In addition to functional particularity, they may form a separate age cohort with associated attitudinal and behavior characteristics. And there is evidence that these junior generalists are moving toward a separate professional identity. See "Associate/Assistant Administrators form Professional Groups: Health Care Management Association of Massachusetts," *Hospital Management* 3 (1971), 34.

*Chapter 6*


# THE ADMINISTRATOR'S PROBLEMS WITH
# ROLE PARTNERS


In order to survive, every institution must obtain key resources from its environment. For the health facility the
most common resource is money: money is used to buy
economic goods and services which are converted into output
(patient care and service). This output is a basic unit of
exchange which the facility offers potential clients in return
for resources they hold.

In the health facility, the office principally responsible for
effecting the exchange of output for resources held outside
the institution is the health care administrator. His duties are
to supervise and coordinate the services and procedures that
form the output and to ensure that each operational unit has
sufficient supplies of resources to complete its tasks. In turn
the administrator also negotiates and facilitates the exchange
with clients. He keeps records of what is sold and what is
coming to the institution; he attempts to iron out difficulties

that arise and impair the exchange; and he is responsible for keeping the overhead costs (that is, the amount of resources consumed by the administrative process) at a minimum.

If we look at the separate administrative offices as collectively composing a network or system, we see that the administrative system forms the institution's infrastructure: the offices and procedures through which resources are continuously being collected and distributed throughout the institution. Viewed from this perspective, the network of administrative offices forms a resource extracting, processing, and allocating system in which individual administrators perform various tasks.

In order to provide patient services, the health institution must buy drugs, food, linens, and equipment; hire and pay the salaries of dietitians, aides, nurses, clinicians, and clerical personnel; pay utility bills. Most of these funds are drawn from patients through charges for services provided and material consumed. These charges, in turn, are often passed along by the patient to his insurance plan, Medicare, Medicaid, or other third party. The institution's administrative cadre is responsible for determining costs, preparing the patient's bill, and collecting the reimbursement. Once the reimbursement is received, it sees to it that money is exchanged for labor, utilities, equipment, materials, and other resources which the operating units of the institution utilize in performing their tasks and providing their particular services for the next patient.

As we have seen above, the individual administrator is pressed by a number of conflicting demands as he carries out the exchange activities. Many of these conflicting demands or expectations come from those the administrator must engage while extracting or allocating resources. This is because those who possess or control resources are themselves the objects of expectations to which they must conform; expectations that cause them to attempt to control the behavior of others in order to reduce stress and strain on themselves. Thus, the

Medicare administrator expects the health care administrator to be patient, quiet and understanding while he slowly and carefully reviews the claim, tends to other business, and, overall, looks out for the interests of his own offices while the medical staff members of the health facility expect "their" administrator to process reimbursement claims as quickly as possible so that resources they want can be obtained. So on the one hand, the health care administrator is expected to be patient, understanding and quiet while on the other hand, he is expected to be aggressive and principally concerned with getting "things" for his own institution. What does the "good" administrator do when confronted with such contradictory, mutually exclusive sets of expectations?

## Resolving Role Conflicts

There is a sizable empirical literature recounting the stresses and strains that characterize the modern health care facility, especially the general hospital.[1] Unfortunately, there is no systematic summary of this descriptive material which can serve as a basis from which to extract a set of hypotheses concerning the sources and resolution of role conflicts. In the absence of such hypotheses, we shall offer a theoretical model of conflict resolution. From this model future research hypotheses might be formulated.

Dahrendorf[2] illustrates the origins and theoretical resolution of role conflict in a model based on the notion of the degree of sanction associated with the alternative expectations. He differentiates among *must-expectations,* which are sanctioned by law, *shall-expectations,* which are sanctioned by specific organizations or institutions (being dismissed from a position or excluded from an association for violation), and *can-expectations,* which are entirely positive in nature (doing a volunteer act—canvassing for the Red Cross—which results in increased esteem for the doer).

Dahrendorf suggests that since an actor is capable of distinguishing levels of sanctions (for example, legal penalty versus peer disapproval), he will select the expectation reinforced by the greatest positive, or the least negative, sanction. This is a useful, if rather obvious, observation, one which is probably confirmed more often than not. But Dahrendorf's mini-max construct does not help us understand how actors resolved conflicting expectations based on similar sanction levels; nor does it provide the basis for comprehending behavior when the more heavily sanctioned expectation is rejected (for example, young American draft resisters). In an effort to augment Dahrendorf's work, we shall offer the following formulation.

We find a beginning point for further analysis in the hypothesis drawn from the work of Gross, et al.[3] that interrole and intrarole, intersanction-level and intrasanction-level conflicts (e.g., shall/shall, must/shall expectations) will be resolved after weighing three factors: (1) the actor's perception of the legitimacy of each expectation; (2) sanctions likely to derive from nonfulfillment of each expectation; and (3) the actor's moral or ethical orientation.

Some actors will constantly seek to avoid the greater negative, or to secure the larger positive, sanction. Such an actor, possessed of this "expedient" orientation, would refuse to participate in a strike or walkout in support of a staff union *if* he perceived that such a violation of an institutional personnel policy would result in a negative sanction—such as dismissal or letter of reprimand. (The intriguing and fundamental question here is: How does the actor come to decide that the institution's sanction is likely to be forthcoming or that the organization's negative response outweighs the increased prestige he might receive from the union by demonstrating support of it?) Seeking constantly to maximize advantage, the expedient administrator's goal is to survive, and, by surviving, to prosper.

A contrasting type of conflict resolution is the "formalist" orientation. Here the actor will, regardless of sanction, base his behavior on what he deems legitimate. Faced with illegitimate and legitimate alternative expectations, the formalist will always reject the former; when two alternatives are offered and neither is seen as illegitimate, the formalist will select that which most closely approximates his own notion of what is proper; and when confronted by two alternatives he considers illegitimate, the formalist will ignore them both. Rectitude, rather than approval or advantage, is the formalist's cardinal principle.

Our conceptualization of administrative behavior, predicated as it is on the actor's perception of the demands made on him and the type of sanction that might be employed to reinforce them, provides the frame of reference for discussing the problems that the administrators mentioned with various offices and bodies both in and outside the health care facility. The model conceptualizing administration as essentially the tasks of extracting and exchanging resources, combined with the theory of role behavior as representing the resolution of various demands and expectations placed before the individual administrator, leads to the hypothesis that the health care administrator is required to interact with specific offices and agencies which control or possess resources. These actors place demands on the administrator which are at variance with his own and other role partners' expectations. Because these demands are reinforced by the resources controlled by the role partners, conflicts arise. Operationally, these conflicts are reported as "problems" with specific role partners.

In the following discussion, *role partner* refers to specific offices or bodies which the health care administrator engages in a resource exchange transaction. In the administrator's work, he must deal with a large number of different role partners because in the modern health care industry resources are compartmentalized—there is a high level of occupational and departmental specialization.[4] Medical treatment cannot be obtained from one physician; there is a host of specialists and each is called in, depending on the particular situation to be treated. The same is true for laboratory analyses, clerical services, or plant maintenance. Technically, each actor within this complex organization with which the administrator deals is a role partner. When several actors share possession of the same resource, or are linked together so that they are interdependent, they form a *sector*. Thus the administrator's technical or clerical subordinates are a sector; physicians form a sector; staff organizations are a sector; and so forth. In our analysis we shall analyze role partners at the sector level of generalization.

## Subordinates

Far and away the most frequently cited source of problems for the health care administrator is his subordinates. The resources held by this sector include information (both technical, such as medical records, and the informal but invaluable assessment of "how things are going" which administrators and co-workers utilize all the time), services, legitimacy (workers confirm that the facility is an "all right" or a "bad" place by their actions and opinions, thereby either attracting to or repelling from the facility other possessors of resources), and even status (if top-rated employees or elite units are employed by an institution, their prestige may be converted into research grants, gifts, and attractions for other high-rated personnel the institution wishes to recruit). It is no wonder, then, that 64% of the respondents volunteered that supervising and evaluating subordinates created major problems; and 28.8% reported that recruiting or training subordinates troubled them.

These data and the comments of respondents reveal a major difficulty confronting the administrator. His superiors claim the right to evaluate him against the performance of his unit, which means on the performance of his subordinates. But, typically, the criteria or performance standards of the superior are not spelled out. At the same time, subordinates, both individually and collectively, present the administrator, usually covertly but occasionally directly, with their own expectations as to what they consider "reasonable" criteria that he should employ in evaluating them. Of course the administrator has his personal notions, derived from observing other units, from his formal studies, or presented to him through professional organizations that serve as reference groups. Whose expectations should be given priority?

## Staff Organizations

Organizations composed of health care personnel offer a particular set of problems to the administrator. One aspect is that while all *organizations* possess economic goods and services, information, prestige, legitimacy and the potential for force in their own right, the *individuals* who comprise them also control vital resources. The American Nurses Association, for example, has considerable resources at its command which can be turned against an administrator—for example, in a contract bargaining situation. But the staff nurses themselves can augment the resources of the Association by withholding their services, broadcasting negative assessments of the institution, or by *threatening* to strike, thereby individually and collectively bringing coercion against the administrator.

Another problem caused by staff organizations is the dissimilarities in their methods of employing their resources in support of their demands. In the automotive industry, representatives of the various unions sit down with representatives of management and ultimately arrive at a contract. This is not so in the health industry. Physicians' and nurses' associations eschew joint collective bargaining; these high-status professional organizations not only ignore but vigorously condemn the organizations of "lesser" occupations. The style and rhetoric of the American Medical Association and the

American Federation of State, County, and Municipal Employees, or the Services Employees International Union, are as different as the life styles, values, and attitudes of the two distinct classes from which their members come: each pursues its own self-interests, but the two refuse to formalize their mutual interests through joint collective bargaining.

Where once the only powerful trade unions with which the health administrator had to deal were the AMA and the ANA, the 1960s witnessed an expansion of unionization down through the hierarchy of the health care professionals. Also the nature of the issues which came to occupy the attention of many staff organizations changed.

The American Nurses Association has moved to a much more aggressive stance in attempting to overcome the low wages, job insecurity, and disadvantageous working conditions found in the hospital. The California Nurses Association and several other state-level organizations have begun collective bargaining with facility administration and seem to be fully committed to traditional organized labor procedures —including strikes.[5] In many California hospitals the CNA has signed contracts establishing "Professional Performance Committees" which are analogous to the shop grievance committee in other industries. The committees not only bring nurses' representatives and management together to discuss the firing, promoting, and scheduling of nurses, they also discuss matters associated with the quality and procedures of patient care.[6]

Along with the rise of militant nurses' associations,[7] the health care administrator finds that other workers are organizing. Medical interns,[8] radiologic technologists,[9] hospital pharmacists,[10] and maintenance employees,[11] among others, are asserting their claims for higher wages, improved working conditions, and job security by agreements that establish recruitment and promotion criteria that amount to "closed shop" agreements with their employers. The results of this professional collectivism for the administrator are constantly evolving relationships with role partners, new actors with which to deal, conflict and confusion within the ranks of the occupational groups arising from some individuals resistance to being involved in "trade-unionism," rising labor costs, and the necessity of becoming quickly skilled in "human relations" and "labor negotiations" techniques. The acute care short term administrator has not been the only one to find himself surrounded by staff associations and labor organizations: administrators of psychiatric hospitals,[12] health maintenance organizations,[13] and Veterans Administration facilities [14] have watched their workers unionize.

If the issues involved were purely economic, hospital labor relations would be complex enough. While improving salaries is one issue involved in most labor disputes, money is not typically the sole—even the major—point of contention.[15]

Demands for increased pay, better working conditions, and formalization of hiring and firing policies often have at their root the belief that the facility is victimizing and exploiting its employees—that is, that the semiprofessionals and unskilled workers are being mistreated because they are largely minorities and women. To a large degree, the success of unionization is related to the growing awareness of racism and sexism on the part of employees, *and* the ability of organizers to combine economic and social reform issues in their organizing appeals. For example, observers of the campaign to organize New York's largely Black nonprofessional health care workers note that the organizers used issues, organizing techniques, and even personnel from the civil rights movement.[16]

Many commentators on the rise of militant nurses' organizations have linked the nurses' rejection of the passive dependent role in the hospital to the challenge to sexist exploitation and discrimination throughout the society. For example, Virginia Cleland calls sex discrimination the nurse's most pervasive problem.[17] Joan Roberts and Thetis Group liken the exploitation and discrimination of women in hospitals to that of Blacks in American society.[18]  Barbara and John Ehrenreich remark: "As health workers, women occupy subservient and underpaid slots: 70% of the nation's health care workers are women, but only 7% of the nation's physicians are women."[19]

Linking sexism and racism as Roberts and Thetis and others have done is important to the understanding of the complexity of human relations and interoccupational group frictions which arise in various ways to bedevil administrators. As Table 23 reveals, although males comprise about one-third of the "health technologists and technicians" category, their median salary is 42% greater than their female peers. In the technologist and techinician category, Blacks are

Table 23

Relationship of Sex and Ethnicity to Income and Occupation in

Hospitals[1]

|  | Total | | Blacks | |
| --- | --- | --- | --- | --- |
|  | Males | Females | Males | Females |
| Health Technologists & Technicians |  |  |  |  |
| 1970 Total | 80,000 | 184,000 | 8,000 | 16,000 |
| Median Income | $7,368 | $5,182 | $6,932 | $5,252 |
| Health Service Workers |  |  |  |  |
| 1970 Total | 143,000 | 1,077,000 | 37,000 | 233,000 |
| Median Income | $4,425 | $3,265 | $4,595 | $3,682 |

1
 United States Bureau of the Census, Statistical Abstract of the U. S. (Washington, D. C.: Government Printing Office, 1973), Table 375.

employed in a proportion approximately equal to their numbers in the overall workforce. But note that the Black male median salary is nearly 32% greater than that of the Black female.

In the less prestigious, less well-paying "health service workers" category, males account for only 11% of the group; but, apparently, they are singularly fortunate or exceptionally well-prepared since their median salary is 36% greater than their female co-workers.

Not only are women disproportionately found in this bottom stratum, but Blacks are also. While Blacks constitute about 10% of the overall workforce, Black males constitute 25.9% of all health service workers and Black females 21.6%. And as in the case of the Anglos, the males receive a higher median wage than the females. (The fact that Blacks in this category make as much as Anglos may be attributed to the concentration of Black service workers in metropolitan areas such as New York, Chicago, and St. Louis where not only the wage rate but also the cost of living is higher than in the thousands of town and city facilities throughout the Mid-West, East and West which chiefly employ Anglos.)

Along with improving economic situations, many staff organizations, especially nurses' associations, are attacking the traditional inferior status and self-image of female health care workers. In a very large measure, this drive against sexism is a generational phenomenon with young women who bring their attitudes and demands about civil rights, anti-war, and feminist causes from the college campus into the hospital or clinic. Wessen unintentionally provides an illustration of both the generational and sexism aspects in his observation of the problem a senior staff nurse had with a student nurse. In a role-playing exercise designed to indoctrinate the student nurse into the mores of the health care industry, the senior nurse is asked to explain why she has instructed the students to stand aside at doorways and allow the physician to enter first. Isn't this a reversal of customary protocol, asks the student? Yes it is, replies the instructor, but it is done to signify the respect paid the physician by the nurse because "they contribute more to the community" than does the nurse and thus are due this act of respect.[20]

Along with the growing concern about racism and sexism, some staff organizations are beginning to pressure administrators to reform patient treatment procedures and standards. Often this pressure is reinforced by direct confrontation coupled with the use of coercion—that is, the threat to strike. The Student Health Organization and the Medical Committee for Human Rights, among other organizations, have employed these tactics. During the summer of 1973 the National Physicians' House Staff Association, a body comprised of interns and residents, included along with a demand for increased salaries the demand that the hospitals correct poor conditions and inferior patient care. In a clear investment of coercion, the president of the NPHSA stated the case: "The quality of professional services is a negotiable issue. As a physician, I cannot be required to work under inferior conditions." An arrangement was subsequently signed with Los Angeles' county-run hospitals.[21]

In addition to considering the militancy, expansion, and lack of integration of staff organizations, we should not overlook the fact, discussed in the previous chapter, that many professional associations perform an accreditation function. As we saw, accreditation, aside from representing potential withdrawal of legitimacy, costs the administrator a good deal of time because of reports which must be prepared. On-site visits also consume the administrator's time as well as strain his nervous system.

Surely no individual administrator would find himself beset by all the problems that staff organizations potentially can create. Nevertheless, one-third of the sample agreed that staff organizations such as professional associations or unions cause them problems. This figure should be seen in the context of the problems reported with subordinates (and nurses and physicians, as we shall see in the following sections). Some recruitment and training problems could well stem from licensing, accrediting, and seniority provisions and procedures established by organizations. Kovner summarizes the effect on staff organization thusly: "The problems of the administrator increase with the number of bargaining units and the number of unions in any one hospital."[22]

## Physicians

It is commonplace for discussions of health administration to deal at length with the conflicts between the administrator and the physician. Some have stressed that this conflict arises from the physician's resentment toward the administrator for interfering in the "sacred doctor-patient relationship."[23] A less hyperbolic explanation rests in sociological and social psychological lore: the administrator is essentially a johnnie-come-lately professional without much status in the industry or prestige in the community, while the physician has expertise, prestige, status and legitimacy among patients and in the community.[24] Another analysis of the roots of administrator/physician conflict places emphasis on the modes of control open to each. The administrator's power rests on an impersonal hierarchy of command, reinforced by the formal sanctions of the institution. He gains compliance by manipulating the symbols of institutional authority. Distinct from this essentially bureaucratic mode of control is that of the physician which rests largely on his technical expertise. He performs the most needed service—treatment of the patient. And he gains compliance not by relying on institutional sanctions but his technical competence and position at the peak of the health care industry's pyramid of professional prestige. Thus, conflict arises because of the competition and confusion which develops when neither can successfully subdue the other since their authority is based in two different domains.[25]

Whether or not there is in fact a "dual authority" pattern of exclusive jurisdictions, or whether there needs to be such a situation, is largely moot. Conflicts that cannot be ascribed to other causes are blamed on dual authority—the would-be health care administrator is assigned to read materials that report its existence; the physician is led to believe that he should attempt to preempt administrative control in some areas and to challenge it in others. Thus, dual authority takes on the characteristic of a self-fulfilling prophecy: it is believed to exist, thus it has consequences for those who do not question its existence.[26]

From the point of view of our role expectation, resource exchange model of administrative behavior, the physician is a role partner of the administrator because he is a major (if not exclusive) source of certain resources that the administrator must obtain. The physician manipulates his resources in an attempt to force the administrator to conform to the physician's expectations and demands for administrative behavior. In this regard, the physician is no different from other role partners encountered by the administrator.

The power of the individual physician and the medical staff is derived from the range and quality of resources possessed and their significance for the health facility. The administrator is at a marked disadvantage because, acting as broker of the facility's resources, he lacks control of resources which are as vital to the physician's well-being as the physician's are to the facility's. The imbalance in the physician/administrator exchange and the leverage this gives the physician becomes apparent when we examine the resources the physician has at his disposal.

The American system of health care grants to the physician nearly exclusive control of the technical skills of diagnosis, prescription of treatment, and surgery—that is, the major income-producing patient services.

Because the physician has been able to claim nearly exclusive jurisdiction in decisions involving patient treatment, he has also gained a monopoly over medically important information. He records much of the patient's data and has control over the contents of the patient's medical file. In addition, by restricting the dissemination of technical information to medical school classrooms, and by obscuring communications in almost unintelligible jargon, the physician controls access to and the availability of technical information about curative and diagnostic procedures and practices.

While writers from the era of the Greek Middle Comedy through Molière and down to George Bernard Shaw were able to exploit the medical men as comic material by characterizing them, as they were seen by their societies, as money-grubbing, ineffectual pedants who mumbled Latin while ministering, bleeding, and purging,[27] the prestige of the physician has been dramatically increased in the twentieth century. In part through artful public relations, in part by largely successful efforts by the AMA to establish some minimal code of ethics and standards of competence, and in part because Americans have come increasingly to equate wealth with social importance, the contemporary physician receives a very high level of esteem and deference from his community.[28]

Because of his technical expertise, information, and prestige, the physician holds a virtual monopoly of legitimacy in making decisions concerning patient treatment. Within his domain, which is largely self-defined, the physician is generally thought to be properly in control. This control means that while some physicians will personally reject one colleague's procedure for another, other physicians will refuse to interfere or publicly to brand ·the man incompetent.

On his sizable deposit of resources the physician earns a special dividend: coercion. Coercion is the ability to threaten the flow or acquisition of other resources needed by the institution. By denying or withdrawing information, services, legitimacy, or prestige, the physician clearly jeopardizes the continuing operation of the facility. When he overtly or covertly *threatens* such a withdrawal, the physician is investing coercion to secure his aims. Because the administrator lacks commensurate control over access to the facility, this being effectively held by the medical staff, he has no equal store of threat to neutralize that of the physician.

While we have concentrated on the imbalance which exists in the power relations of administrators and physicians, we can substitute any other health care office for the administrator and see a similar situation. Vis-a-vis the nurse, for example, the physician is clearly stronger because he controls quantities of resources she cannot match. The same is true with the board of trustees or its equivalent. While it is true that *individual* physicians may be replaced or sanctioned by trustees because trustees may withdraw staff privileges or cancel the house physician's contract, this power evaporates in the face of the collective resources of the medical staff or, as we have just seen, an organization of physicians such as the National Physicians' House Staff Association.

Why, then, does the health care administrator have a difficult time controlling the physician or exercising control in areas in which the physician claims jurisdiction? It is not because of the physician's sacred trust, or his greater contribution to the community, or his expertise. It is rather because the physician is able to marshall more resources than the administrator and withhold almost at will resources the institution must obtain in order to survive, and because the resources at the disposal of the administrator are less important, less crucial to the maintenance of the physician's interests than the converse. Consequently, the physician has enormous leverage with the administrator. The same is true for other relationships of which the physician is a part. The physician dominates the nurse or aide or technician not because he is the "top professional"; rather he is the "top professional" because he commands resources required by his co-workers or which (like prestige or coercion) can be spent to secure the physician's interests. If a physician claims a particular nurse is incompetent, he is placing not only his legitimacy, information, and prestige on the table against her, but also his implicit threat of withdrawing his resources from the institution unless his demands are met.

In light of this assessment of the power bases of the physician it may seem paradoxical to suggest that his power is *decreasing.* In fact, I believe this is the case. For one thing, the body of physicians is becoming more heterogeneous in attitudes and values. Younger physicians are much less prone than their older colleagues to follow the lead of senior members or the AMA. General practitioners, interns, residents, academically affiliated physicians, researchers, public health doctors, and various board-certified specialists are increasingly becoming aware that many of their interests are not those of other subdivisions of the profession. Thus, the physician no longer speaks with the weight of a unified establishment behind him.

At the same time, tasks and responsibilities once exclusively the province of the physician are passing into the hands of nurse practitioners, paramedical personnel, and various technical and clinical groups. This has both grown from and caused the awareness that many of the privileges and prerogatives claimed by physicians may well have been overvalued— that is, the facility can have many services performed by other less expensive (and not only in terms of salary) personnel.

Vis-a-vis the administrator, the physician is still in a powerful position; but as health care administration becomes more bureaucratic and technological, and as essentially administrative skills become more vital to the maintenance of the facility, the position of the administrator is strengthened. It is the growing dependence on administrative skills and personnel that is in large measure responsible for the redefinition of the traditional physician/administrator relationship noted by several observers.[29]

In terms of the resource-exchange model, the value of

several resources held by the physician has declined by the appearance of alternative suppliers; at the same time, the skills and services possessed by the administrator have risen in value. The analogy is suggested by the recent round of monetary reevaluations. While the physician is not likely to be declared bankrupt, he, like the United States in international trade, may find that his currency no longer is worth as much, is no longer the standard unit for calculating value as it once was.

Nevertheless, the physician remains one of the principal role partners of the administrator. This is revealed in the frequency with which the sample mentioned the medical staff (or individual physicians) as a source of problems. Twenty-two percent volunteered that they had major problems from this role partner. Asked if physicians caused them any particular problems, 60.4% replied affirmatively.

When we analyzed the remarks about physicians, we found that demands for special equipment or services, or problems of reconciling conflicts between physicians and other health care workers were commonly cited. Repeatedly, administrators voiced the belief that physicians did not understand the requirements and demands of the institution—that is, the expectations for the behavior of physicians held by the administrator. The inability of the administrator to enforce upon the physician his expectations through effective sanctions appears at the base of many of the administrator's complaints.

### Nurses

Forty-one percent of the respondents affirmed that they had problems with nurses. Of this total, nearly 25% (or 11% of the overall sample) indicated that their problem was their inability to recruit or retain top quality nurses.

The recruitment and retention of nurses, and to a lesser extent other semiprofessional and unskilled workers, involve a complex set of factors. Obviously, the availability of suitably trained candidates is a primary consideration. In many parts of the United States, there are more openings than individuals seeking employment. But in other areas, such as San Francisco, Boston, and Los Angeles, there seems to be either an equilibrium or even a surplus of nurses. Therefore, finding recruits may not be as large a part of the problem as commonly believed.

Retention and turnover of personnel are related to several things, among them the fact that many young women who come out of nursing departments and programs enter the job market fully intending to work for only two or three years. And aside from those who enter the hospital seeing their jobs as only temporary, some proportion of nurses get married, become dissatisfied with the profession or the facility, decide to change jobs or cities, or in other ways choose to leave.

But a good many nurses, married or not, wish to continue working. Indeed, many nurses are the principal or sole providers for their families. Yet some of these individuals who wish to continue to work and who do not intend to change jobs are among those who leave a given facility. Why?

Some leave because they are judged incompetent or incompatible by their supervisors. However, it may be that economic forces are also at play which have a direct bearing on the administrator's difficulty with retaining top quality nurses.

Salaries are a major (as much as 60%) item of hospitals' budgets. In many cases, nurses' salaries account for half the wage budget—that is, as much as 30% of total hospital expenditures. In most facilities, nurses are paid in relation to their "merit"—in fact, usually on the basis of accumulated seniority *in the institution.* By applying economic models of income optimality and the principle of diminishing returns, it is possible to calculate at what point in years of service the individual nurse's improving skills, knowledge of the institution's routine, and so forth, fall below her rising salary line.

Where the efficiency curve and the salary curve intersect is a critical point in time because prior to this point (say during the nurse's first 3 or 4 years) the facility is actually enjoying an optimal return from the nurse's labor in relation to what she is being paid, but after the intersect point, annually increasing salaries make the individual nurse increasingly less attractive *economically*. Because seniority is only accrued in the employing facility and cannot be transferred, it makes economic sense to fire (or effectively force nurses to resign by giving them unattractive schedules or undesired duties) an individual nurse for the reason that with other facilities following the same policy the pool of unemployed but experienced nurses is rather large. And even if an experienced individual cannot be found who will take the opening (and lowest) pay scale, the facility actually remains ahead financially if it employs a rookie.

There is some evidence that nurses are aware of this practice and concerned about job security. In a study of striking nurses in Cleveland, Ohio, job security, communications with the administration, and the hospital's hiring and firing policies were seen as the major issues.[30]

If this speculation is correct, then there are several factors related to the turnover and inability to retain or recruit top quality personnel. But the administrator himself may in part be responsible for some of their apparent difficulties. With salaries rising and nurses' associations becoming increasingly militant, *and* with mounting pressures to reduce or hold down costs falling on the administrator, it would seem that economically-based confrontations over hiring and firing policies will become more frequent.

Aside from problems associated with hiring and firing, administrators reported problems with nurses stemming from the former's responsibility for intervening in disputes involving the latter and other health workers or administrative personnel. Many of these problems seem to have their roots in the nature of the expectations nurses derive from their professional associations.

Argyris notes that nurses and physicians, like teachers, lawyers, and other professionals, tend to have a primary bond with their profession rather than with the particular institution at which they work.[31] When conflicting demands are seen in the expectations of the profession and the expectations of the institution, the resolution is made in favor of the former. This disturbs the administrator who, because his professional identification or the expectations of his professional associations are less heavily sanctioned in his eyes, places his primary identification and his primary source of expectations with the institution.

Argyris also suggests that nurses create problems for the administrator because nurses see the administrator as a second-class citizen of the health care society—second class, that is, in comparison to physicians—and release their pent-up frustrations on him.[32] Stripped from its implicitly sexist stereotyping of females as emotional, unstable creatures who "blow their tops," there may be a core of truth in this observation. Nurses may be more hard-nosed in their dealings with administrators than with physicians or other health care workers, not because administrators are "second class citizens," but because administrators are seen as holding fewer resources, and therefore, possessing weaker sanctions than other major role partners upon which nurses must depend to accomplish their duties.

And some fraction of the problems administrators report having with nurses stem from the growing militancy and dissatisfaction with their traditional situations of being underpaid and exploited. Strikes and other labor disputes to which nurses are a party are often expressions of these social and economic concerns.[33]

## Board of Trustees

At the top of the institutional hierarchy sits the board of trustees or its equivalent. Twenty-eight percent of the sample affirmed problems with the board. Typically, these problems arose from requests for special data or reports, the necessity of securing the board's consent for a major allocation of resources such as a plant expansion, or inquiry by a trustee for information about some administrative matter or patient service. It is noteworthy that problems arising from attempts at favoritism or in pursuit of an individual trustee's interest were rarely mentioned. The bulk of problems stem from the board's discharging its responsibility for administrative oversight and financial management.

The primary importance (of the board) to the institution does not rest in its control function, but rather in the role of the board members in securing resources, especially money, for the institution from private and public funders. Secondarily, the board members bring certain technical skills, such as a knowledge of the law, finance, or business methods, to the institution. We see these two functions reflected in the membership of the boards of nonprofit facilities throughout the United States.

In Boston, Berger and Earsy found that "businessmen dominate boards, with lawyers and financiers representing the next most common occupational categories."[34]  In Detroit, Goldberg and Hemmelgarn found that business executives, lawyers, accountants, physicians and hospital administrators control boards.[35]  In Pittsburgh, Elling and Lee report that two-thirds of the members of health care planning boards and boards of trustees were Protestant Republican businessmen.[36]  In a longitudinal study of the composition of a board of a 345-bed nonprofit community hospital in a middle-sized Midwestern city, Holloway, Artis and Freeman reveal that over 50% of the members of the board between 1910 and 1959 were what the authors called "economic influentials"—that is, businessmen and successful professionals.[37]

Individual trustees help connect the institution to the community in which it exists. This function also is performed by the commissioners, directors, or politicians who oversee government facilities. Members of the corporate boards of directors who govern proprietary facilities generally are selected with an eye to the stockholder groups they represent or to the other corporations and economic interests with which they are affiliated. Thus, the trustee or his equivalent forms a link between the organization and important elements of its environment.[38]

Individuals are brought onto boards because of their connections to money, or because the prestige, information, legitimacy, and authority they possess can be used by the institution to secure economic goods and services. Each trustee is expected to contribute one or another resource through his connections to major social, economic, and political institutions and the elites who control them. Conceptualizing the struggle for resources as "the hospital-support game," Elling pinpoints both the resources and the discretionary position of the elite-allocators: "Clearly the elite, especially the industrial, financial, and legal leaders, [are] central in the final channeling of support in one direction rather than in another."[39] Elling goes on to cast his findings in terms of a research hypothesis: "That organization will be better supported than another if the elements in the environment with which it is mainly identified and with which it has the most connections are more dominant than those with which the other organization is identified and connected."[40] What Elling is saying is that institutions with which elites are associated are able to translate the prestige and legitimacy they obtain from membership of elites on their board into cash and other resources held by the community, private foundations, and government agencies.[41]

At one time, the social, economic and political elites themselves sat on hospital boards. This is rarely the case now, except in the smaller communities. A close look at the composition of boards reveals that the members may be economic notables or influentials, but they are not of the ruling class of the community—they are not the owners or

the highest executives of the corporations or the senior
partners of the most prestigious firms. Rather, the board
members are generally of the second tier—they may be the
executives of national corporations or the managers of the
local plants or the confidants of the ten or twenty most powerful men who often are either their business associates or their
lawyers. These men are of the governing class; they conduct
the day-to-day business of the community and are selected
for this role because of their skills. They are aided by the
ruling class insofar as skills, ambition, and ability is needed to
retain the support (and resources) of their peers and patrons
in the various economic and political institutions of the
community.[42] It is the emphasis on skills which is largely
responsible for the growing numbers of lawyers, management
experts, and successful businessmen on boards. Being the
scion of an old and distinguished family is no longer the
sufficient criterion for a seat on a hospital board—especially
the board of a large multiservice community hospital or
major medical center.[43]

Looking at the composition of boards and the criteria for
membership, we see several areas of potential conflict with
health care administrators, especially with upper level administrators in charge of facility expansion, community relations,
and fiscal management. Because most trustees come out of
the business world where they have won more than an
average measure of success, they are schooled in business
management techniques and philosophies and view these as
perfectly reasonable criteria for evaluating health care delivery. But the delivery of health care does not admit to
many of the techniques and criteria of the business world:
there is no basic unit of output as there is in industry or
commerce. There is no standard pricing policy—some patients
pay more and some pay less for the same procedure. In
addition performance in the health care industry cannot be
measured in terms of profits: if the bottom line in a business
enterprise is black, good; but does red ink on the hospital's
ledger mean the facility is failing to meet its obligation to the

community? Of course not because good health or the absence of infirmity is generally regarded as an intangible yet first priority to be pursued for its own sake—no economic value can be put on gaining good health. In other words, techniques and practices which would win esteem in the business community may be inappropriate in many hospital situations.

Similarly, the trustee's connections with the external political and economic institutions may bring him into conflict with the administrator who wishes to push past the board a medically sound but politically controversial new program or facility—such as an abortion service, an out-patient clinic in a minority neighborhood, or an affirmative action hiring program. Such confrontations of conflicting positions arise from different reference groups and may be involved in much of the dispute over recognizing unions and engaging in collective bargaining. In communities ruled by elites with a strong anti-union bias, it would be unlikely that an administrator who wished to recognize a staff union would be permitted to do so by his board. Such an act of recognition would be interpreted by the business leaders as encouraging their own employees and other unorganized service workers (such as teachers, firemen, municipal workers, and so forth) to unionize—a prospect hardly likely to be favored by the local power structure. Thus, the potentially divergent expectations of the administrator and the trustee offer a range of conflict that will expand with the continuing evolution of health care into a public utility ever-more interconnected with the political and social processes of the community.

Why would a man who is busy with a career of considerable responsibility take on an additional workload of unremunerated service by joining a hospital board or other local health agency? He gains prestige, certainly, and legitimacy in the community. He is seen as performing a public service, a civic duty. From among all those who might serve, he is chosen—he is one of the "anointed."[44]

Looking beyond these symbolic rewards, we discover

dividends to trustees in the form of information and authority: information about expansion plans, the investment patterns of the institution, and other activities in the community which may be released at board meetings or as a result of contacts with other elites resulting from their mutual membership. Authority is the right to speak in the name of the institution. Here it refers to the ability to allocate the institution's resources by setting and controlling policy. This competence may be used to reward friends or to keep rewards away from enemies (as in the letting of contracts to suppliers, builders, and equipment vendors). In any event, it will be used to increase the individual's own sense of self-worth and quite possibly his prestige in the community. Such memberships are part of the conditions one must meet to become and to remain a "local notable"—a publically recognized local or regional elite.

For some individuals, membership on a hospital board is an opportunity to demonstrate their executive skills and ideological reliability. The ambitious, seeking to rise in the governing class and to be recruited into more important positions in government or the economy, use occasions such as those presented to trustees to showcase themselves. This may mean attracting the attention of conservative businessmen by being toughminded and tightfisted, or winning recognition from liberal community leaders, politicians, or labor leaders by supporting new managerial or technical procedures and "rationalization" of the health care industry.

While demonstrating managerial expertise, the trustee also has an opportunity to show his political skills, his ability to work under the pressure of competing demands. And, of course, the trustee is in a position to demonstrate his commitment to the basic assumptions of the ruling class: that the existing social and economic institution must be preserved at the least possible cost to them through accommodation and reform. The trustee has an opportunity to illustrate his acceptance of this necessary pre-condition of entry into the higher levels of the institutions controlled by the ruling class when he supports fee-for-service, traditional hierarchical management privileges and practices, efficiency models of institutional evaluation, economic incentives (and sanctions) to manipulate and control employees, and other procedural/organizational prerequisites of the contemporary social and economic system. Because the health care industry is a nexus linking the local community, various governmental levels, and major economic institutions, hospital boards, committees, and commissions offer an unsurpassed opportunity to launch careers and promote personal and group interests.

The fact that few administrators are troubled by trustees suggests the ability of local notables and other elites to conduct their affairs well beyond the workaday environment of most administrators. This suggests a parellel between the board/facility and elite/community relationships. The general hypotheses drawn from community power studies might act as guides for further consideration of the style and significance of board behavior. Alford has summarized the findings of community studies thusly:

1. Public decision-making at any specific time occurs within a relatively narrow "agenda of alternatives" determined by constraints of political and economic structure and culture;
2. When working-class groups are organized into politically active unions, a base of opposition to the middle class is created which allows the raising of a variety of issues not usual when only the middle class is active.
3. Many major decisions are made autonomously by the private economic leaders and are not subject to public control.[45]

## Patients

We have seen that dealing with patients accounts for 7.1% of the administrator's average day and that 39.6% of the sample reported a problem with determining costs or charges for patient services. It comes as no surprise, therefore, to find that 64% of the respondents affirm that they had problems with patients or their families.

While we did not explore this issue, it is reasonable to suspect that the source of many of these problems is the inability or unwillingness of the patient to conform to the administrator's (or another health worker's) expectations. It is one of the anomolies of the health care industry that those for whom it exists are often bossed and bullied, belittled and degraded into conforming to the providers' demands. The obvious resolution of this apparent contradiction is that health care institutions do not exist for the patient; the institution exists for the physician, the health care worker, and the health care administrator, and is gracious enough to provide room for the sick and injured who have little to say about what they receive since they, unlike the previously mentioned, have nowhere else to go. Because administrators and providers view the average patient as being unable to exercise sanctions in support of his demands on health care providers, there is little or no compulsion to modify their behavior to conform to the patient's expectations.

After all, the average patient does not control any resources: his bills are paid, whether he is pleased or unhappy with the service he receives, by insurance companies and government agencies; or if he lacks coverage and is medically indigent the facility itself covers the services. Courts and credit bureaus stand ready to reinforce the institution's demands for payment from recalcitrant patients by adding their sanctions (which tend to be considerable—must and shall sanctions, respectively) to those of the institution. But when the patient is well endowed with resources (particularly money, however prestige weighs heavily), special consideration is taken and, as Duff and Hollingshead have shown, health care providers and administrators significantly change not only their own behavior (thus responding to the patient's expectations of them) but also permit the patient considerable leeway in his own deportment: providing special diets, disregarding established visiting hours, scheduling procedures to conform to the patient's timetable.[46]

There are indications, however, of a struggle underway to

redefine the patient's position in the health care industry. Consumer protection is currently fashionable and a wide range of organizations, including the Medical Committee for Human Rights, Health-PAC, and the NPHSA, among others, are attempting to use their resources to compel changes. The *Darling* decision and other recent court cases have increased the scope of liability and degree of responsibility of the facility for the quality of patient service. Convalescent hospitals that once all but escaped inspection and regulation are subjected to new and more demanding standards of care; in part as a result of pressures from insurance carriers concerned about malpractice suits, in part from government out of concern for rising costs, and in part from within the industry in order to avoid further government action.[47] While the individual patient remains largely defenseless, the patient as a social role is taking on new allies who may introduce new resources to back up the patient's demands.

## Variations by Occupational Category

Table 24 indicates that frequency of problems with role partners varies with occupational category. Or to put it differently, some partners are much more significant to the incumbent in one administrative office than another.

As we have been led to expect from previous profiles, convalescent hospital administrators stand apart and have a substantially independent set of problems with role partners. For instance, neither medical staffs nor trustees are reported as sources of problems. The former is easily explained: convalescent hospitals do not employ residents, interns, or house physicians; consequently, there is no medical staff to give the administrator problems. In the same manner, trustees, at least as the office exists in general hospitals, do not exist. All the convalescent hospitals in the sample are proprietary institutions with ultimate executive authority held either by the owner-administrator or by a corporate body. Since several of the institutions in the study are part of multi-institution

Table 24

Problems with Selected Sectors by Occupational Category

| Activity | Convalescent Hospital Adm | Chief Adm Short Term & Extended Care Hospital | Department Adm | Administrative Assistant | Outpatient Clinic Adm | Total Sample |
|---|---|---|---|---|---|---|
| "What major problems do you have to deal with...?" | (Percent Mentioning) | | | | | |
| Subordinates (Supervising & Evaluating) | 41.2 | 59.1 | 76.7 | 69.6 | 33.3 | 64.0 |
| Subordinates (Recruiting & Training) | 58.8 | 13.6 | 39.5 | 8.7 | 0 | 28.8 |
| Medical Staff | 0 | 40.9 | 14.0 | 34.8 | 33.3 | 22.5 |
| "Do you have a problem with...?" | (Percent Affirming) | | | | | |
| Physicians | 70.6 | 63.6 | 51.2 | 73.9 | 33.3 | 60.4 |
| Nurses | 58.8 | 45.4 | 37.2 | 43.5 | 0 | 41.4 |
| Staff Organizations, Unions, or Associations | 23.5 | 40.9 | 27.9 | 39.1 | 50.0 | 33.3 |
| Board of Trustees (or Equivalent) | 0 | 40.9 | 23.3 | 43.5 | 33.3 | 27.9 |
| Patients or Their Family | 70.6 | 86.4 | 51.2 | 60.9 | 83.3 | 64.0 |
| Total Number of Cases | 17 | 22 | 43 | 23 | 6 | 111 |

chains owned by large corporations, the local administrator would be responsible, in a manner somewhat similar to that of the nonprofit facility administrator to his board, to the corporate management. To believe that no problems arise between the site administrator and his corporate superiors calls forth an uncommon degree of credulity.

Recruiting and retaining nurses and other employees was a problem more frequently mentioned by convalescent hospital administrators. Since the services provided by such facilities are narrower than in other sectors of the industry and are much more dependent on nurses, aides, and maintenance personnel, it is logical that the staff they employ would be the major concern and the primary source of problems to convalescent hospital administrators. Lower salaries, higher staff/patient ratios, and lower occupational prestige for convalescent hospital workers may also give rise to confrontations with administrators.

The division between administrators with specific operational responsibilities (department administrators) and administrative generalists (chief administrative officers and administrative assistants) that we noted in the profiles of their activities and problems reappears again on Table 24. Subordinates are the most likely role partners to cause problems for department administrators, and less frequently cited as causing problems by the two generalist categories. All other role partners are more frequently cited by CAOs and AAs than by DAs.

I suspect that the variation between line and staff administrators' frequency of citing problems with subordinates is derived from the fact that DAs are more likely than AAs to have large numbers of subordinates on their immediate work team. Some department administrators oversee 40 or 50 (or more) individuals; administrative assistants rarely supervise more than half a dozen. Moreover, the DAs are responsible for a number of complex procedures, many of which involve clinical or technical procedures or direct patient care services.

The possibility of conflicts with subordinates increases proportionately. The subordinates of most AAs, however, typically are clerical personnel or administrative support staff such as accountants, auditors, or legal advisors. Thus, both the smaller number of subordinates and the nontechnical, nonpatient care services that these workers perform would work to reduce problems with subordinates. At the same time, the more integrative and comprehensive scope of the chief administrative officer's and the administrative assistant's duties would bring them into far more contract with physicians, nurses, and patients than would the more insular department administrator.

### Size and Type of Facility

Administrators of small (proprietary) facilities and their colleagues from large (mostly governmental) institutions apparently are less likely to have problems with their medical staffs or boards than are their colleagues in 200 to 699 bed (nonprofit) institutions. Table 25 suggests that size is associated with greater frequency of problems that are related to supervising and evaluating subordinates and staff organizations. This may reflect the fact that the larger facilities also are governmental institutions. As Table 26 shows, administrators of government facilities report a much greater frequency of problems with organizations. In the Veterans Administration facilities the administrator not only must deal with the U.S. Civil Service Commission but also with the American Federation of Government Employees which enrolls VA employees.

Among the three size categories which are primarily composed of administrators from nonprofit facilities, (100-199, 200-399, and 400-699 beds), increased size is associated with increased problems with boards of trustees and, perhaps, increased frequency of problems with subordinates. Increased size, as we noted, associates with both occupational and departmental specialization which, in turn, are factors that

Table 25

Problems with Selected Sectors by Size of Facility

| Sector | No Beds | 1 - 99 Beds | 100-199 Beds | 200-399 Beds | 400-699 Beds | 700 & more Beds | Total Sample |
|---|---|---|---|---|---|---|---|
| "What major problems do you have to deal with...?" | | (Percent Mentioning) | | | | | |
| Subordinates (Supervising and Evaluating) | 25.0 | 46.7 | 63.2 | 66.7 | 80.0 | 77.3 | 64.0 |
| Subordinates (Recruiting and Training) | 12.5 | 40.0 | 31.6 | 14.8 | 40.0 | 31.8 | 28.8 |
| Medical Staff | 37.5 | 13.3 | 31.6 | 33.3 | 20.0 | 9.1 | 22.5 |
| "Do you have a problem with...?" | | | | (Percent Affirming) | | | |
| Physicians | 25.0 | 80.0 | 78.9 | 44.4 | 70.0 | 54.5 | 60.4 |
| Nurses | 87.5 | 53.3 | 57.9 | 55.5 | 25.0 | 40.9 | 41.4 |
| Staff Organizations, Unions, or Associations | 37.5 | 26.7 | 31.6 | 22.2 | 35.0 | 54.5 | 33.3 |
| Board of Trustees (or Equivalent) | 25.0 | 0 | 10.5 | 37.0 | 60.0 | 13.6 | 27.9 |
| Patients or Their Family | 100.0 | 80.0 | 68.4 | 63.0 | 60.0 | 50.0 | 64.0 |
| Total Number of Cases | 8 | 15 | 19 | 27 | 20 | 22 | 111 |

Table 26

Problems with Selected Sectors by Type of Facility

| Sector | Proprietary | NonProfit | Government | Total Sample |
|---|---|---|---|---|
| "What major problems do you have to deal with...?" | (Percent Mentioning) | | | |
| Subordinates (Supervising and Evaluation) | 40.9 | 64.8 | 80.0 | 64.0 |
| Subordinates (Recruiting and Training) | 45.5 | 18.5 | 34.3 | 28.8 |
| Medical Staff | 13.6 | 33.3 | 14.3 | 22.5 |
| "Do you have a problem with...?" | (Percent Affirming) | | | |
| Physicians | 72.7 | 55.6 | 60.6 | 60.4 |
| Nurses | 63.6 | 40.8 | 34.3 | 41.4 |
| Staff Organizations, Unions, or Associations | 27.3 | 25.9 | 51.4 | 33.3 |
| Board of Trustees (or Equivalent) | 0 | 33.3 | 31.4 | 27.9 |
| Patients or Their Family | 77.2 | 72.2 | 48.6 | 64.0 |
| Total Number of Cases | 22 | 54 | 35 | 111 |

contribute to communications, technological, and personnel management difficulties.

When we compare the 100-199 and 400-699 bed columns, we find a marked difference in frequency of problems with several role partners. Boards of trustees are more frequently mentioned by respondents from the larger institutions, as are problems with subordinates. Nurses and the medical staff are less frequently cited by these same administrators.

The range of services and the magnitude of expenditures characteristic of the smaller facilities probably explain why their administrators report fewer problems with trustees and subordinates: fewer complex requests go before the board; less diversity and fewer jurisdictional barriers arise resulting in a smaller probability of finding malcontents and "characters" on the staffs of the smaller institutions. In the larger institutions, there are probably as many or more types of problems and certainly more occasions for these problems to arise, since there are more nurses and medical staff members as well as greater specialization of administrative responsibility. There are more administrators in a large facility, some who may have no contact at all with nurses and physicians, and others who may have specific jurisdiction in medical staff disputes; therefore, the overall administrative cadre in larger facilities may report a lower aggregate profile of problems because the larger staff number reduces the average frequency.

Moving to the gross comparisons of proprietary, nonprofit, and government administrators, we encounter several basic differences. The "government" column of Table 26, which reflects the responses of administrators largely drawn from extended care unifunctional facilities, reports lower levels of problems with patients and medical staffs than the nonprofit column which is composed of administrators from short term, general hospitals and HMOs. The government administrators, however, have a lower rate of subordinate problems and problems with staff organizations.

The frequency of reported supervising and evaluating problems increases significantly from proprietary to nonprofit to government administrators; confirmation of problems with nurses declines in the same direction.

When we compare the profiles of the government and proprietary administrators with that of the nonprofit administrators, we find that in matters of medical staff and physicians, the two unifunctional categories stand below and above, respectively, the multifunctional. This may reflect the absence of house staffs and a reliance on a few resident physicians backed up with private physicians who have staff privileges. Since extended care government facilities and convalescent hospitals provide mainly residential and rehabilitory services rather than medical or clinical procedures, they depend on their dieticians, aides, orderlies, and maintenance personnel for survival. This is reflected in the significantly higher frequency with which respondents from unifunctional institutions complained about problems of recruiting and training subordinates.

Within the overall sample, subordinates are the most frequently cited source of problems. The conflict results because the administrator's superiors judge him on the performance of his subordinates, and while the subordinates have their own expectations of how things should be run, the administrator has his own criteria for the functioning of a professional institution. Whose expectations should be fulfilled?

One-third of the sample cite staff organizations as causing them problems. Because the members of these groups control economic goods and services, information, prestige, legitimacy, and other vital resources for the functioning of the facility, their sanctions include the possibility of withholding their services, broadcasting negative assessments of the institution, or threatening to strike. Also, the fact that they shun collective bargaining denies the administrator a common forum for conflict resolution. During the 1960s unionization of health professionals expanded and these groups became increasingly militant. They began to battle against institu-

tional racism and more recently, against sexism. Some staff
organizations have begun to pressure administrators to improve patient treatment and quality standards. Moreover,
many professional associations perform an accreditation
function. Loss of accreditation would cause the withdrawal
of legitimacy from the facility. Hence, the number of problems for the administrator increases with the number of staff
organizations in the facility.

When asked if physicians caused particular problems,
60.4% of the sample answered affirmatively. The roots of
physician/administrator conflict are based in the distinct
modes of control open to each. The physician controls
several resources the administrator must allocate in the
facility. Because the administrator lacks control of resources
which are as vital to the physcian's well-being as the physician's are to the facility's, there is an imbalance in the
physician/administrator exchange. This gives the physician
tremendous leverage with the administrator. Many respondents claimed that physicians did not understand the
requirements and demands of the institution. Specifically
they cited problems due to demands for special equipment or
special services, or with reconciling differences between
physicians and other health workers.

Problems with patients or their families was affirmed by
64% of the sample. The source of these problems is the
unwillingness or inability of the patient to conform to the
administrator's expectations. The patient is viewed as controlling few resources; therefore, the facility has little in-
centive to modify its behavior according to the patient's
expectations. Recently the consumer protection movement
has begun to use its resources to compel changes. Thus, while
the individual patient is relatively defenseless, the patient as a
social role is acquiring new allies whose resources may help to
implement the patient's demands.

It was found that the frequency of problems with role
partners varied with occupational category. Again the convalescent hospital administrator's profile was distinct. For

him medical staffs and trustees are not reported as problems, while recruiting and retaining nurses and other employees are more frequently cited. The DAs profile indicates that subordinates cause the majority of their problems. All other role partners are cited more frequently by CAOs and AAs than by DAs.

Problems also varied according to size and type of facility. Administrators of the small and large facilities apparently have fewer problems with their medical staffs and boards than those of the middle-size institutions. The extended care, unifunctional facilities report fewer problems with patients and medical staffs than the nonprofit hospitals. Respondents from unifunctional institutions had more complaints about problems of recruiting and training subordinates.

# NOTES

1. C. Argyris, *Diagnosing Human Relations in Organizations: A Case Study of a Hospital* (New Haven: Yale University, Labor and Management Center, 1965); T. Burling, E. M. Lentz, and R. N. Wilson, *The Give and Take in Hospitals* (New York: G. P. Putnam's Sons, 1956); S. H. Croog, "Interpersonal Relations in Medical Settings," in H. E. Freeman, S. Levine, and L. G. Reeder (eds.) *Handbook of Medical Sociology* (Englewood Cliffs, N.J.: Prentice-Hall, 1963), 241-271; R. S. Duff and A. E. Hollingshead, *Sickness and Society* (New York: Harper & Row, 1968); B. S. Georgopoulos and A. Matejko, "The American General Hospital as a Complex Social System," *Health Services Research* 2 (1967), 76-112; B. S. Georgopoulos and F. C. Mann, *The Community General Hospital* (New York: Macmillan, 1962); L. G. Jackson, *Hospital and Community* (New York: Macmillan, 1964); A. R. Moss, et al., *Hospital Policy Decisions: Process and Action* (New York: G. P. Putnam's Sons, 1966); C. Perrow, "The Analysis of Goals in Complex Organizations," *American Sociological Review* 26 (1961), 854-866; M. I. Roemer and J. W. Friedman, *Doctors in Hospitals: Medical Staff Organization and Hospital Performance* (Baltimore: Johns Hopkins Press, 1971).

2. R. Dahrendorf, *Essays in the Theory of Society* (Stanford: Stanford University Press, 1968), 39-41, 49-52.

3. Cf., N. Gross, W. S. Mason, and A. W. McEachern, *Explorations in Role Analysis* (New York: John Wiley, 1958).

4. Many of the critics of the health care industry argue that the apparent compartmentalization is actually fragmentation, and that fragmentation is one of the principal causes of the poor quality and often unavailability of care. The solution these critics offer is the "rationalization" of the system, a process that seems to mean the "planning" of facility construction, the bringing of services together in regional medical centers so as to reduce duplication while taking advantage of alleged economies of scale, and the application of "business" principles and practices as criteria for evaluating delivery of care and making executive decisions. See the discussion of the "corporate rationalizers" in R. R. Alford, "The Political Economy of Health Care: Dynamics Without Change," *Politics and Society* (1972), 127-164. Defenders of the "cottage industry" style of American health care usually view compartmentalization as "pluralism." They defend the system as insuring the consumer a wide range of types and styles of services—from private solo practitioners through prepaid group plans to small proprietary hospitals and major medical centers. For example, M. Halberstam, "In Defense of the System," in R. H. Elling (ed.) *National Health Care: Issues and Problems in Socialized Medicine* (Chicago: Aldine-Atherton, 1971), 89-107; H. Schwartz, "Health Care in America: A Heretical Diagnosis," *Saturday Review* 54 (14 September 1971), 14-17, 55.

5. N. K. Grand, "Nursing Ideologies and Collective Bargaining," *Journal of Nursing Administration* 3 (1973), 29-32.

6. E. H. Erickson, "Collective Bargaining: An Inappropriate Technique for Professionals," *Nursing Forum* 10 (1971), 300-311.

7. B. Bullough, "New Militancy in Nursing: Collective Bargaining Activities by Nurses in Perspective," *Nursing Forum* 10 (1971), 273-288.

8. See the discussion of the National Physicians' House Staff Association in the *Los Angeles Times* (4 December 1973).

9. D. L. Barnes, "Collective Bargaining for Radiologic Technologists," *Radiologic Technology* 45 (1973), 79-89.

10. A. J. Hidde and T. R. Covington, "American Society of Hospital Pharmacists View Collective Bargaining," *American Journal of Hospital Pharmacists* 30 (1973), 428-435.

11. J. Shinn, "How Local 1199 Wins Over Hospitals: Soul Power, Black Power, and $120.76 a Week," *Modern Hospital* 116 (1971), 39-42. Also see Health Policy Advisory Center, "Health Workers," a packet of four Health/PAC *Bulletins* (March 1970; July-August 1970; April 1972; November 1972).

For a detailed history of Local 1199 and an account of the strike against New York hospitals, see E. Langer, "Inside the Hospital Workers: The Best Contract Anywhere," *New York Review of Books* 16 (20 May 1971; 3 June 1971), 25-33; 30-37. Also see J. and B.

Ehrenreich, "Hospital Workers: A Case Study in the 'New Working Class,' " *Monthly Review* 24 (1973), 12-27.

12. R. M. Health, "The Role of Union and Management in Public Psychiatric Hospitals," *Journal of Mental Health Administration* 1 (1972), 15-22.

13. "5,000 Hospital Workers Win New Contract," *Service Employees* 33: 8 (February 1974), 2. An account of a successful strike at 14 clinics and 11 hospitals of the Kaiser Foundation of Northern California.

14. The American Federation of Government Employees is the principal organizer of VA employees. See A. R. Somers, *Hospital Regulation: The Dilemma of Public Policy* (Princeton: Princeton University, Industrial Relations Section, 1969).

15. J. S. Rakich, "Hospital Unionization: Causes and Effects," *Hospital Administration* 18 (1973), 7-18; D. D. Pointer and N. Metzger, "Work Stoppages in the Hospital Industry: A Preliminary Profile and Analysis," *Hospital Administration* 19 (1972), 9-24; D. D. Pointer and H. Graham, "Recognition, Negotiation, and Work Stoppages in Hospitals," *Monthly Labor Review* 94 (1971), 54-58.

16. B. and J. Ehrenreich, *The American Health Empire: Power, Profits, and Politics* (New York: Vintage, 1971), 238-239.

17. V. Cleland, "Sex Discrimination: Nursing's Most Pervasive Problem," *American Journal of Nursing* 71 (August 1971), 1542-1543.

18. J. I. Roberts and T. M. Group, "The Women's Movement and Nursing," *Nursing Forum* 12 (1973), 303-322.

19. B. and J. Ehrenreich, *The American Health Empire*, 237.

20. A. F. Wessen, "Hospital Ideology and Communication Between Ward Personnel," in E. G. Jaco (ed.) *Patients, Physicians, and Illness*, 2nd. ed. (New York: Free Press, 1972), 331.

21. *Los Angeles Times* (4 December 1973).

22. A. R. Kovner, "The Hospital Administrator and Organizational Effectiveness," in B. S. Georgopoulos (ed.) *Organization Research on Health Institutions* (Ann Arbor: University of Michigan, Institute for Social Research, 1972), 366.

23. Burling, Lentz, and Wilson, *The Give and Take in Hospitals;* H. L. Wilensky, "Dynamics of Professionalism: The Case of Hospital Administration," *Hospital Administration* 7 (1962), 20; G. Bugbee, "Administration and the Professional in the Hospital," *Hospital Administration* 6 (1961), 26-33.

24. Georgopoulos and Mann, *The Community General Hospital*, 567.

25. W. V. Heydebrand, *Hospital Bureaucracy: A Comparative Study of Organizations* (New York: Dunellen, 1973), 193 and passim; W. R. Scott, "Professionals in Hospitals," in B. S. Georgopoulos (ed.) *Organ-*

*ization Research on Health Institutions* (Ann Arbor: University of Michigan, Institute for Social Research, 1972), 156; F. L. Bates and R. F. White, "Differential Perceptions of Authority in Hospitals," *Journal of Health and Human Behavior* 2 (1961), 262-267.

26. H. L. Smith, "Two Lines of Authority: The Hospital's Dilemma," in E. G. Jaco (ed.) *Patients, Physicians, and Illness*, 1st. ed. (New York: Free Press, 1958), 468-477; *Modern Hospital*, symposium issue, "Doctors and Hospitals" (January 1969).

27. See R. Boxill, *Shaw and the Doctors* (New York: Basic Books, 1969).

28. R. Stevens, *American Medicine and the Public Interest* (New Haven: Yale University Press, 1971). On the role of the AMA in expanding the physician's power base in the local community and also with the political system, see "The American Medical Association: Power, Purpose and Politics in Organized Medicine," *Yale Law Journal* 63 (1954); R. Harris, *A Sacred Trust* (New York: New American Library, 1966); E. Cray, *In Failing Health: The Medical Crisis and the AMA* (Indianapolis: Bobbs-Merrill, 1970); J. Furrow, *AMA–Voice of American Medicine* (Baltimore: John Hopkins Press, 1963).

29. See Jackson, *Hospital and Community;* P. J. Gordon, "The Top Management Triangle in Voluntary Hospitals," *Journal of the Academy of Management* 4 (1961), 205-214.

30. Grand, "Nursing Ideologies," 32.

31. Argyris, *Diagnosing Human Relations* 62.

32. Ibid., 67-69

33. J. A. Alutto, "The Professional Association and Collective Bargaining: The Case of the American Nurses Association," in M. F. Arnold, L. V. Blankenship, and J. H. Hess (eds.) *Administering Health Systems: Issues and Perspectives* (Chicago: Aldine-Atherton, 1971), 103-126.

34. I. Berger and R. Earsy, "Occupations of Boston Hospital Board Members," *Inquiry* 10 (1973), 43.

35. T. Goldberg and R. Hemmelgarn, "Who Governs Hospitals?" *Hospitals* 45 (1971), 72-79.

36. R. H. Elling and O. J. Lee, "Formal Connections of Community Leadership to the Health System," *Milbank Memorial Fund Quarterly* 44 (1966), 294-306.

37. R. G. Holloway, J. W. Artis, and W. E. Freeman, "The Participation Patterns of 'Economic Influentials' and Their Control of a Hospital Board of Trustees," *Journal of Health and Human Behavior* 4 (1963), 88-99. There is, however, a noticeable trend toward managerial and technical expertise, rather than mere social distinction, among the elites selected for membership.

38. J. Pfeffer, "Size, Composition, and Function of Hospital Boards of Directors: A Study of Organization-Environment Linkage," *Administrative Science Quarterly* 18 (1973), 349-364.

39. R. H. Elling, "The Hospital-Support Game in Urban Centers," in E. Freidson (ed.) *The Hospital in Modern Society* (New York: Free Press, 1963), 104.

40. Ibid., 106.

41. Cf., L. V. Blankenship, "Power Structure and Organizational Effectiveness," in R. Presthus, *Men at the Top: A Study in Community Power* (New York: Oxford University Press, 1964), 368-404; L. V. Blankenship and R. H. Elling, "Organizational Support and Community Power Structure," *Journal of Health and Human Behavior* 3 (1962), 257-269; I. Belknap and J. Steinle, *The Community and Its Hospitals* (Syracuse: Syracuse University Press, 1963).

42. The ruling class is composed of the 2% or 3% of the population that either controls or owns outright the major economic institutions. The governing class includes the holders of major elected political offices, senior administrators of public agencies, and official or informal advisors of these officeholders. See G. W. Domhoff, *Who Rules America?* (Englewood Cliffs, N.J.: Prentice-Hall, 1967); F. Hunter, *The Community Power Structure* (Chapel Hill: University of North Carolina Press, 1953).

43. L. E. Bellin, "Changing Composition of Voluntary Hospital Boards: An Inevitable Prospect for the 1970s," *HSMHA Health Reports* 86 (1971), 674-681.

44. The term is Hacker's. See A. Hacker, "The Elected and the Anointed: Two American Elites," *American Political Science Review* 55 (1961), 539-549.

45. R. R. Alford, *Bureaucracy and Participation: Political Cultures in Four Wisconsin Cities* (Chicago: Rand McNally, 1969), 194. See the brilliant review of community power research and its bearing on public policy formation and execution in J. Walton, "The Bearing of Social Science Research on Public Issues: Floyd Hunter and the Study of Power," in J. Walton and D. E. Carns (eds.) *Cities in Change: Studies on the Urban Condition* (Boston: Allyn & Bacon, 1973), 318-332.

46. Duff and Hollingshead, *Sickness and Society*.

47. See L. McCoy, "Licensing of Nursing Home Administrators," *Medical Care* 9 (1971), 127-135; W. W. Rogers, *General Administration in the Nursing Home* (Boston: Cahners, 1972).

*Chapter 7*


# STRENGTHENING HEALTH CARE ADMINISTRATION


The picture of the health administrator which emerges from the preceding pages is that of a college-educated individual who has risen within the health care industry to his present position. He comes to this post from a nonclinical, nontechnical background, but with previous administrative experience. His overall high level of involvement in the profession of health care administration is reflected in his membership in several professional associations and his regular reading of two or three trade journals or professional periodicals. Charged with the responsibility of securing and managing the goods, services, and other resources which the health care institution needs for survival, the health care administrator spends most of his time communicating with selected role partners. These communications are often efforts to resolve problems undermining the effective allocation of resources. Outstanding topics and subjects with which problems are encountered include budgeting and financial

management, services operating at a loss, Medicare, regulations and laws, and difficulties which the administrator has
with medical equipment and management technology. Subordinates, physicians, and patients or their families occupy
much of the administrator's time and are related to most of
the problems he deals with. In negotiating with his role
partners, the health care administrator is frequently at a
considerable disadvantage because he commands fewer
resources of value to his partner than vice versa. Many of the
problems with which the health care administrator must
grapple arise from this vulnerable bargaining posture—a
posture which strains the administrator because of the conflicting demands he receives from partners and sectors whose
sanctions weigh heavily on him. Even sectors or partners less
endowed with resources than the administrator, such as the
patient, create problems because the administrator cannot
readily compel them to adhere to his expectations and demands for their behavior.

The administrator's relationship with his role partners is
dynamic and evolutionary. These changes are spawned or
exacerbated by complex economic, social, and political
forces such as innovations in medical and managerial technology, the continuing growth and strengthening of professional reference groups, and the increasing bureaucratization
of medical care delivery. These forces thrust new problems
and conflicts upon the administrator and reinforce existing
ones.

The administrator himself is aware of his problem and has
some notions about how to prepare himself to cope with
them. It seems that one of the reasons for the overall high
levels of involvement with professional associations and trade
publications is the desire to see what other administrators
and observers of health care administration have to say about
current problems and trends. The workshops he attends and
articles he reads are largely problem-oriented: they aim to
help the serving administrator execute his extraction/
exchange tasks more successfully.

Apparently many health care administrators look to higher education for help. During the informal presurvey discussions with health care administrators about their professional problems and the ways this research might be used to illuminate them, several administrators inquired about the courses and programs being offered at the principal investigator's university. From these conversations it became apparent that an interest existed in continuing education. Implicitly, and often explicitly, health care administrators indicated that they sought to upgrade their skills or obtain new ones, or were merely curious about what was going on in college classrooms. In an effort to see what administrators were interested in, the respondents in the survey were asked: "If you had the time and opportunity, are there any college subjects or courses you would like to take that you think would enable you to do a better job?" Table 27 presents a summary of their replies.

## In-Service Training

The courses which administrators feel would be useful to them largely reflect the major problems and activities which engage them. These include courses in accounting, personnel management, organization and methods, and similar administration subjects. The administrators were asked if there was a specific orientation or departmental identity for the administration courses. Courses dealing with hospital or health care administration were more frequently cited than business administration.

Advances in medical technology and management tools, especially the increased utilization of computers, is evidently much in the minds of many health care administrators. They want to learn more about the applications and procedures involved in technological innovations. Their concern with technology goes beyond administrative applications and is reflected in their interest in courses dealing with medical technology and techniques.

Table 27

College Subjects Sought by Health Administrators

| Course or Subject | Times Mentioned |
|---|:---:|
| Administration | |
| Business Administration | 7 |
| Health Care Administration | 7 |
| Hospital Administration | 18 |
| Management Tools | |
| Computer Technology & Data Processing | 7 |
| Systems Analysis | 5 |
| Communications and Human Relations | |
| Reporting Procedures and Patterns | 12 |
| Communications Skills (Public Speaking, Writing, etc.) | 4 |
| Human Relations | 6 |
| Labor Relations | 6 |
| Public Relations | 2 |
| Medical and Technical | |
| Medical Technologies & Techniques | 6 |
| New Medical Trends | 3 |
| Community Health Planning | 4 |
| Specific Patient Care Services (Aging, Alcoholism, Outpatient, etc.) | 8 |
| Nursing | 2 |
| Social Science | |
| Psychology | 15 |
| Sociology/Social Welfare | 9 |
| Anthropology | 2 |

Aside from learning new processes or procedures, many administrators want to improve their ability to deal with people. Making reports and learning how to utilize information within and between components of the health industry as well as more narrowly and traditionally defined courses such as English composition and public speaking, and human, labor and public relations drew interest. Given the wide range of role conflicts with which the administrator is beset, it is not surprising that many respondents mentioned psychology and sociology as subjects they felt would help them do a better job.

Admittedly, we must be cautious in drawing too much from these expressed preferences. It is one thing to tell a college student interviewer that a given course would be useful; it is quite something else to go out and take it. Be this as it may, the preferences of the respondents are so closely associated with what we found to be their major activities and problems that we believe they reflect genuine interests, even concerns, on the part of many health care administrators. After all, individuals who received a top-flight educational preparation with sound schooling in administrative procedures as well as an introduction to medical technology and techniques (which probably *excludes* most liberal arts and science majors) would find little resemblance between the classroom examples and many of their current problems. Educators from health care administration programs admit weaknesses in their instruction when they repeatedly call for reforms in curricula and the incorporation of new experiences to make health care administration "relevant."[1]

The conclusion seems inescapable: in-service, mid-career training and education will strengthen the health care administrator and improve his ability to carry out his duties. In other words, making the latest academic and professional information available to administrators will reduce overhead costs by upgrading the institution's infrastructure.

This upgrading is neither quickly nor easily accomplished. To increase the health care administrator's stock of economic goods and services, prestige, or authority would require a major reallocation of existing stocks, a reallocation we are sure will not take place because those who presently hold these resources simply cannot be induced to surrender them. But it would be relatively easy to increase the administrator's store of technical information and administrative expertise. If he improves his skills, the health care administrator will be even more valuable to his facility. As his value to the institution and the industry rises, so will his standing in the community of health workers and in the overall society. Increased technical skill and increased prestige allows the health care administrator to assert his jurisdiction and his authority in matters once considered beyond the proper sphere of his control. Relationships with his role partners will be redefined; and these redefinitions will earn dividends in the form of increased coercion. With a growing supply of coercion in his hand, the administrator in effect has a dividend earned by his other resources—a dividend which can be invested to earn compound interest.

## Areas of Instruction

If we were analyzing health care administration from the point of a human relations model of administration, or from the perspective of its place in the evolution of the delivery of medical care, we should see the administrator's problems and activities quite differently than we have. By setting the health care administrator in the context of organizational maintenance, and then conceptualizing the function of the office as managing the extraction and allocation of resources required by the institution, we place emphasis on the technical and social-psychological aspects of an essentially economic enterprise.

This model mmmmmmmmmmmmmmmmmmmmmmmmmmmmmm

role of the health care administrator as administrator, not as a health care worker. To be sure, the administrator must be familiar with the basic structures and processes of the industry, just as the school administrator or the prison administrator must be informed about the idiosyncrasies of his industry. But the central emphasis must be on administration, not its setting.

Because our research has revealed distinctive patterns of activities, problems, and role partners associated with occupation, size, and type of facility, we won't attempt to develop detailed curricula here. Some specialization is desirable, especially at the postgraduate or in-service levels. For instance, convalescent hospital administrators and administrators of extended care government facilities such as mental or psychiatric institutions need particular preparations which would be replaced with other programs for administators of short term facilities. And outpatient clinics, to return to a sector too long ignored in this study, may form another separate group for instructional purposes.

We have seen that the health care administration profession is highly fluid: individuals move around a good deal, both from job to job within an institution and from institution to institution. Regardless of their institution or occupation, however, they work with a fairly narrow range of sectors: patients, physicians, nurses, technical and clerical subordinates, community groups, political and government agencies, staff organizations, third party payers. The health care administrator needs to know the resources these sectors contain and the typical expectations the sectors have for themselves and for health care administrators. To take just one example, the administrator must know how to keep abreast of the regulatory and legal constraints imposed on his sphere of the institution. This does not mean he must know the conditions himself; rather, he must know where to turn in order to keep minimally current *and* where to turn for quick and accurate information when it is needed. Knowing the institution's major resource sectors, what they hold, and what they expect is the equivalent of knowing the "rules of the game" or the "decision rules" which game theoretists and simulation experts are so fond of emphasizing.

Learning the institution's and his office's decision rules is characteristic of the basic need to be able to think abstractly and to communicate both his thinking processes and conclusions to others. A practical application of abstract thinking is found in the routine planning exercises the administrator is called upon to perform. Budgeting, inventory control, program development and subordinate evaluation are common activities which rely on the ability to think abstractly.[2]

In order to free himself from the crush of routine chores, the health care administrator must be able to converse comfortably with the computer. He must know how and when to use it as well as its limitations—especially the implications for the quality of interpersonal relations resulting from relying on computers to arrange information profiles. Computers are very careful and tidy but completely insensitive to the idiosyncrasies and special requirements of human beings.

We have seen that the scope of governmental intervention in the health care industry creates major problems for many administrators. And while it is beyond the present study to document, it is clearly the case that this intervention is growing. It is also taking new forms, such as Professional Standards Review Organizations, new Medicare accounting and reporting requirements, comprehensive health planning, and affirmative action investigations. At the same time, both the quality and quantity of health care have become major political issues. Exposes, investigations, sit-ins, and direct confrontations with individual facilities are becoming increasingly common. Attitudes of indifference to and passive acceptance of the legitimacy of health care providers are changing to much more aggressive demands for accountability—for example, witness the spiralling rise in malpractice suits. It is not an overstatement to claim that the environment within which the administrator works is heating up and becoming less benign, and that one of the principal agents of this change is the contemporary political system.

Where once the administrator could meet his civic obligations through either his nonprofessional volunteer activities or his efforts to educate the community to its health needs, he can no longer avoid direct engagement in the political processes which envelop the hospital. The administrator has always been a major political actor because of the resources which his institution holds; but now he must address other political forces and actors which he formerly either ignored or which simply did not exist. Moreover, his task is complicated because many of the new political actors and issues grow out of social and economic institutions and processes of which he is only slightly aware and understands even less—such as institutional racism or sexism.

In the present context it seems appropriate to stress the utility of gaining insights into contemporary social, economic, and political forces and institutions through social psychology, sociology, political science, and economics—especially the economics of nonprofit organizations. With the rapid evolution of the health care industry, characterized by its central stage position in American politics, much of the philosophy and many of the procedures encountered in business administration curricula are of increasingly marginal applicability to the health administrator, even if he is on the proprietary side of the industry. While many lower and middle level administrators can increase their efficiency and effectiveness by obtaining technical training in bookkeeping, operations research, personnel management, and other traditional areas of business, the upwardly mobile and more responsible members of the profession will need the understanding of the political processes and social forces which is presented throughout sociology, political science, and public administration courses.

You will recall that the overall community from which our sample was drawn is multiethnic. In thinking over the problems administrators encounter with subordinates and with patients, I wonder how many of these time-consuming situations grew out of the situation of a middle-class Anglo male dealing with a nonmiddle-class, non-Anglo individual. Sociologists have repeatedly confirmed that class, sex, and ethnicity are major correlants with differential attitudes and behavior. When these three factors come together in an individual relationship which must be conducted in the inherently stressful conditions of a hospital or other health facility, can we reasonably expect that misunderstandings and conflicts will not be proliferated?

Problems arising from insensitivity and ignorance are not going to be eliminated because, like illness, they are part of the human condition. Yet just as the frequency and severity of illness can be reduced by intelligent timely action, so can the problems which stem from the inherent dissimilarity of administrators and many of their role partners decrease. Some remedial effects can be realized through human relations and sensitivity training. And more prevention is available from the hiring and promoting of minorities. The minority administrator can perform two very different yet interrelated services: one is to help reduce tension and misunderstanding by bringing his own knowledge of his role partner's attitudes and experiences into the exchange process. This is not to assume that any woman or any Black will be aware of and sensitive to the needs and expectations of all women or all Blacks with which they must deal, but it can be assumed that the overall probability of this occurring is greater with a minority than with an Anglo male. The second contribution to the institution of minority administrators is their potential as teachers—teaching the institution's staff about the needs of their brothers and sisters. Given the opportunity and the support of their superiors, most minority administrators will volunteer to their colleagues how to reduce cross-communal conflict. Often minority people are placed in offices to appease their community, to show "do-gooders" that the institution is "a responsible citizen," and to allow their superiors the opportunity to congratulate themselves for doing "something progressive." In such a situation, the facility generally expects the minority to "take care of business" involving his (or her) "people." From the facility's point of view, this wastes the important dividend resulting from employing minorities in administrative positions: the possibility of nonminority administrators and members of the staff learning from their minority colleague, learning the needs and expectations of major role partners, and learning how to reduce and avoid expensive conflicts.

These recommendations about the in-service education of health administrators are based on the belief that the individual who happens to serve the facility cannot divorce his civic or humanitarian role from his professional one. The individual's professional role now must incorporate a responsibility to his community that is far more complex than merely "taking the lead in teaching the community about its health needs." The administrator must be aware of the current social, economic, and political waves and currents and must see his actions as part of the overall reality they form.

The old paradigm[3] of administration which sought to distinguish fact from value and insisted that the proper sphere of the administrator was the former is in disrepute.[4] Nazi Germany, Vietnam, and Watergate illustrate the moral bankruptcy of slavishly following administrative procedures and refusing to consider the social consequences of action. Efficiency, effectiveness, and survival of the institution are important goals and correct criteria for judging and being judged; but they are secondary to moral and ethical obligations one human being owes his fellow human beings.

The current reordering of relationships and redefinition of the place and significance of health care has created massive problems for serving administrators. Nevertheless, the present challenge to orthodoxy and tradition contains the opportunity as well as the need for defining a new paradigm, not just for the health administrator but for all administrators. In working towards this goal we must begin by seeing how and why to separate questions of social equity from production, justice from effectiveness, and reason from loyalty. No one knows the full measure of the new paradigm, but it surely incorporates the requirement that first and foremost the administrator is a member of a community that will hold him accountable for his actions and for those of the institution in which he serves.

## The Health Institution: Focus of Training

Traditionally, students are trained in classroom, examined, and awarded degrees. Once they are graduated, they rarely return to the classroom. Education is seen as a once-in-a-lifetime innoculation with a lifetime warranty against failure or obsolescence. The folly of this notion is nowhere better revealed than among the responses of the present sample of health care administrators. Although most are highly educated, many lack the skills or knowledge to meet the demands of their position.

The distinction between the classroom and the workroom is both incorrect and impractical. It reflects the guild mentality that should have died out with the end of feudalism. And it deprives both the student and the worker from enriching each other through sharing each others' knowledge and experience. This separation is being bridged and can be closed.

Internships and practicae take the student to the institution. The first allows the individual student to become familiar with the role of the institution, its personnel, and its decision rules. The practicum allows teams of students and practioners to work together on one or more actual administrative problems facing an institution.[5]

Significant educational experiences can be provided for mid-career personnel, either on campus or at their institution. There is absolutely no reason other than obstinacy that prevents an institution from contacting individuals with the relevant experience and from offering seminars in administrative and other procedures during working hours. Alternatively, employees can be encouraged to attend evening courses, weekend retreats, and short-term workshops. Already General Motors and other large organizations have training programs for their personnel which approximate middle-sized colleges both in the numbers of enrollees and the scope of courses offered. Such in-house programs can be offered by larger institutions and smaller facilities can pool their support and personnel for such activities.

If equal emphasis is placed on the administrator's social and professional responsibilities, such in-service educational experience will strengthen not only the institution but the profession and the society it serves.

## NOTES

1. See the section entitled "Education for Health Services Administration," *American Journal of Public Health* 50 (1970), 982-1022; M. F. Arnold, "Education for Administration of Health Services," *Public Administration Review* 31 (1971), 537-542; J. D. Thompson and G. L. Filerman, "Trends and Developments in Education for Hospital Administration," *Hospital Administration* 12 (1967), 13-32.

2. See R. Westfall, "Educating for the Future," *Hospital Administration* 16 (1969), 81-94.

3. "Paradigm" is the universally recognized scientific achievements which *for a time* provide model problems and solutions to a community of practitioners. See T. S. Kuhn, *The Structure of Scientific Revolution* 2nd. ed. (Chicago: University of Chicago Press, 1970), viii and passim.

4. For an excellent analysis of the passing of the old administrative paradigm, see V. Ostrom, *The Intellectual Crisis in American Public Administration* (University: University of Alabama Press, 1973).

5. One form of a practium involves ten to twelve students and two to three professors joining with counterparts in a health facility to work on a problem facing the facility. The academic members bring the

theories and procedures from the classroom into operational situations. For example, a planning model can be used to assess the costs and benefits of expanding the facility's physical plant. Working with their professors, students collect data, discuss needs and interests with workers and facility personnel, and prepare a detailed analysis. A report is made to the top administrators and executives of the facility who are encouraged to criticize the effort. From the experience the facility gains what amounts to an extensive professional consultancy; the students gain invaluable experience in a health institution, familiarity with the personnel and services of health care, and an opportunity to practice their skills and have their shortcomings pointed out by professional administrators.

*Chapter 8*

## SUMMARY AND CONCLUSIONS

We have found that significant differences exist among health care administrators of different categories in how they spend their time, the problems they encounter, and the role partners they deal with. At the same time, there are variations among categories in type of academic preparation, level of educational attainment, career patterns prior to and after entering health care administration, involvement in the profession, and such demographic characteristics as age and sex. These characteristics vary according to facility size and type of care of service provided. When we compare the present findings with previously published data, several trends are detected. For example, it appears that fewer M.D.s and R.N.s are filling administrative posts than in the past. It also seems that more women are found among the middle and upper levels of hospital administration and that administrative personnel are changing jobs and employers more frequently than before. While there is no previous benchmark from which to measure, it seems likely that problems with staff organizations and unions as well as difficulties arising from governmental rules and regulations are consuming increasingly larger amounts of the administrator's time.

This final chapter concentrates more heavily upon the differences among the four major occupational categories of health care administrators. We have seen that there is considerable variation among them both in terms of the characteristics of their incumbents and the tasks which they are called upon to complete. I believe that differences among occupational categories of administrators will, during the next decade or so, greatly increase—that is, with the continued expansion of the size and the range of services which health delivery facilities provide, the subdivisions of the administrative cadre will become more and more distinctive. Administrators of specialized departments such as physical therapy, housekeeping, the kitchen, the pharmacy, and the laboratory will become more and more technically specialized in order to cope with the procedures and the problems of their subordinates. It is not at all unlikely that many future department administrators will be selected from among the workers who demonstrate superior skills and an ability for leadership; they will be given training (or required to get it elsewhere) to prepare them for careers as administrators.

It is certainly the case that convalescent administrators will increasingly become a highly recognized separate sector. The enactment of Public Law 90-248 requiring state programs for the licensure of convalescent administrators has given impetus to the formulation of educational requirements which reflect the specific patient needs and services provided by convalescent hospitals. The result can only be an increased specialized identification, a growing "professionalism," in this sector.

If this speculation about growing differentiation and specialization is borne out by subsequent events, we can expect to see fewer "administrative generalists" hired into health care administration. Administrative assistants and probably most chief administrative officers will continue to be generalists because of the integrative and managerial skills required by the nature of their positions. But these generalists will increasingly be dealing with administrative subordinates (i.e., department administrators) whose primary identification may remain with their professional or work group, not the facility as is the case with generalists who lack a strong occupational loyalty. Thus we can expect problems of communication, difficulties with personnel evaluation and recruitment, and disagreement over budgetary priorities. At the same time, we can expect a functional if not formal decentralization of authority since the administrative generalist will be compelled to defer to the department administrator in matters touched by technical or occupational considerations.

This trend towards providing paraprofessional and technical employees with administrative tools will be reinforced by the in-service training programs of their trade associations and by academic programs which will expand their traditional course offerings to include courses in the principles and practices of management—as many nursing departments have recently done in order to attract mid-career nurses who wish to obtain either a Master's degree or a certificate in nursing administration. Thus the links in the chain of command will become weaker because they will not be molded in the same forge. We can expect generalists to have greater difficulties with these administrative specialists because of the latter's greater empathy with their professional comrades: they will side with their subordinates more often than would a generalist because the specialist has by training and socialization incorporated the attitudes and expectations of the work group or profession. Specialization within the administrative cadre heightens the possibility of conflict while complicating the processes of control.

This compartmentalization is suggested by the differences among the present four major occupational categories. Because of implications of a trend toward further specialization in health care administration, it may be useful to summarize some characteristics of the four categories.

## Convalescent Hospital Administrator

In the present sample we found that the convalescent hospital administrator is likely to be younger than many of his colleagues in the general hospital: 41% are 35 years and younger. This age profile may be related to the rapid growth of the industry in Southern California because other studies of convalescent administrators point to a much different age pattern. For example, a Detroit area survey of 40 convalescent hospital administrators reports only 25% 39 or younger and 50% (compared with 29.4% in the present sample) 50 years and older.[1] The Detroit pattern appears nearer the national norm: a 1969 survey of 18,390 administrators conducted by the National Center for Health Statistics found 8.4% under 35 years of age, and 44.8% 55 years of age and older.[2] The importance of the age profile is derived from the inverse relationship of age and education. We see this relationship in comparing our younger Southern California sample with the older national one: 58.9% of the former reported no undergraduate degree compared with 72% of the latter. But while the younger administrator is more likely to have some college, his longer prospective career in convalescent administration suggests that he will be seeking, because of the new licensure requirements and other "up-grading" efforts in the industry, both in-service and continuing academic training.

In terms of the other characteristics, the convalescent administrator stands clearly apart. Measured by the number of trade publications read and the number of associations joined in his own sector, the convalescent hospital administrator is much less likely to rank in the upper levels of professional involvement: indeed, only 6% of the sample received the highest rating. (The other categories averaged 18% in this rating.)

The convalescent hospital administrator's distinctive role becomes apparent when we examine what he is called upon to do. For example, he spends 5 times as much time with patients; yet only one-third as much time in staff meetings and one-half as much time with reports as compared with the administrators in the other categories. He has more problems with laws and regulations, especially with Medicare. His frequency of voicing problems with recruiting and retaining subordinates is the highest of the four occupational groups: 59%.

From the national study we find that the convalescent hospital administrator spends a great deal of time doing essentially nonadministrative chores. As Table 28 reveals, he must be a jack-of-all-trades.

Table 28

Percent of Time Spent in Selected Tasks by a National

Sample of Convalescent Hospital Administrators[1]

| Activity | Percent of Time |
|---|---|
| Administering Facility | 58.8 |
| Kitchen & Dietary Work | 12.5 |
| Providing Nursing Care | 7.5 |
| Clerical Work | 6.5 |
| Housekeeping Services | 6.3 |
| Other | 8.4 |

[1]United States Department of Health, Education, and Welfare, National Center for Health Statistics, "Selected Characteristics of Administrators for Nursing Homes: United States, June-August 1969," Monthly Vital Statistics Reports, 20, supplement(14 January 1972), 1-9.

Because of the rapidly evolving nature of the services provided, the growing numbers of elderly and other individuals seeking convalescent care, and the changing patterns of governmental relations, the convalescent industry presents a particularly difficult case for those preparing the next generation of health care administrators. It seems certain, however, that the needs of the sector must be met by accepting the unique demands and work load of the convalescent hospital administrator and by developing training and in-service programs accordingly.

## Chief Administrative Officer

The pattern of career mobility suggested by the biographies of administrators of general acute care facilities is one of vertical, not horizontal, recruitment. Individuals are brought into the industry at lower and middle range positions (e.g., at the administrative assistant rank, or to fill a technical or service position) and are promoted. The result of this pattern is seen in the aggregate profile of the top executive— the chief administrative officer.

He is older than his colleagues in other ranks (41% are 51 years and older), is a career health administrator (64% report all previous jobs in health care administration; 100% report previous health care administration experience), and is active in his profession (36% earned the highest professional involvement rating—twice the number of those in the department administrator and administrative assistant categories).

The CAO deals with problems which, because of their complexity and seriousness, are beyond the scope of his assistants. For example, he is three or four times more likely to report having to deal with planning and supervising the development and maintenance of the physical plant. He is more likely than DAs and AAs to report problems stemming from Medicare; and he reports the highest frequency of problems with patients: 86% of the category affirmed problems with patients and or with their families.

But it would be misleading to conclude that the chief administrative officer need only be a sophisticated and skilled generalist. While communications and human relations skills are necessary for the position, they certainly are not sufficient. They must be complimented with a firm knowledge of the technical and medical side of the facility. This knowledge is needed to interpret the needs and demands of the clinical and medical staffs since it is in his office that matters which cannot be resolved at the departmental level are thrashed out.

While much of this technical expertise in the lore of the hospital and of medicine can be accumulated through years of apprenticeship in the industry, I wonder if the rapid expansion of the numbers of facilities and the dramatic changes in the technical side of health care which mark the past (and presumably the forthcoming) decade allow for this leisurely, haphazard style of preparing top administrators. Asked differently, are there enough seasoned, first rate administrators to go around? And if not, how can we accelerate the production of them?

## Department Administrator

We have previously stated that the department administrator is more likely to have an academic foundation and actual work experience in a health care or related occupation. And, we suggested that in the future more and more often this individual will obtain his administrative preparation from his professional associations and career training programs. This follows logically from the findings that the department administrator often deals with highly complex technical issues. Even if he is assigned to community relations, personnel, or maintenance, he needs more detailed and sophisticated understanding of associated procedures and practices than one who is serving as administrative assistant or associate hospital director.

We see this narrowness and particularity in the department administrator's problem profile. Nearly 21% report problems with inadequate information, a rate five times as great as that reported by the CAOs. And the department administrator has three or four times as high a percent of reporting problems with subordinates. On the other hand, the range of role partners with which the DA interacts appears to be rather limited—at least, the DA reports problems with them less frequently. The department administrator has a 20% lower rate of problems with individual nurses, physicians, trustees, and patients. The frequency with which DAs mentioned problems with the medical staff is one-third to one-quarter that of CAOs and AAs.

## Administrative Assistant

Reflecting the upward mobility which characterizes the segment of the health care industry covered in the present study, the average administrative assistant is younger than his colleagues: 56% of the category is 35 years or younger. And he has a commensurately shorter tenure in his position. The administrative assistant has fewer subordinates to trouble him (the category mentioned troubles recruiting or retaining subordinates far less frequently than any other—approximately 9%).

While the AA handles routine administrative tasks, he seems to have more trouble with technology and equipment (87% affirmed problems with them) and with securing information and data on time (his confirmation rate of 30% is the highest of any category for this problem). These data reflect an essential aspect of his position—preparation of reports and collection of information to assist his superiors in their decision-making.

Being the junior member of the firm, the AA is not assigned many extramural responsibilities: he spends one-half the CAO's and DA's time in activities which are related to his job but which take place outside of the facility. Nor is he much involved with problems related to Medicare and other governmental regulations or with certifying and licensing

bodies. These tasks are left to the more experienced individuals who occupy higher positions in the hierarchy of
administrative control.

Social scientists are often guilty of distorting the very
phenomenon they are intent on revealing because they abstract their subject out of its social and economic context. To
a large degree, we have committed this error here by concen-
trating almost exclusively on the administrator's perspective.
We have seen much of the conflict and most of the activities
which form the environment within which he carries out his
central purpose of extracting and allocating the resources the
facility needs for survival; but we have only begun to discern
the vague contours of the institutions and forces which give
shape and substance to the administrator's activities.

Before concluding our discussion, I would like to take a
moment to mention what I see as some of the institutions
and forces beyond the immediate circle of the administrator's
interactions. It is in reacting to these externals that the
administrator's environment is largely decided.

1. *The politicization of health care.* Government's role in
delivering and guaranteeing high-quality, readily available
care is expanding. The slogan "health care is a right!" is
clearly the operative premise of most governmental bodies;
while some agencies or bodies may act more aggressively and
progressively, health care is now a de facto public utility. The
demand for health care, both created by other social and
economic programs and stimulated by America's rising
standard of living, will not diminish; if anything, we can
expect the demand to increase as more and more people live
longer and longer. With increased demand comes increased
costs; with increased costs, increased direct and indirect
governmental expenditure and concern, increased governmental regulation and control—either negative (through
licensure) or positive (by making funding available only to
those who accept government guidelines).

2. *Consumerism.* A correlative of the expanding role of

government is the growing involvement of consumers in the affairs of the health care facility. Government has decreed that consumers' representatives shall be part of health care planning bodies. At the local level, consumers' organizations have called for and are receiving membership on hospital boards. On an individual level, the facility can no longer expect its patients to submit meekly to institutional authority; now questions are being asked about costs, about procedures, about the quality of treatment. The professional mystique is being challenged by consumers who demand to know the facts: facilities who refuse are often engulfed in controversy. Consumer organizations are also pressing to gain admission to lay membership on professional licensing boards.[3]

3. *The struggle against racism and sexism.* Across our society there are ample manifestations of concern about and dedication to the fight against racism and sexism. While the intensity of the fight and the battlefields change, we can expect the effects of the conflict to involve health care administrators for years to come.

4. *Unionization.* The organization of health care workers into collective-bargaining units is a manifestation of the reorganization which is taking place throughout American society. Once the extended family, the place of work, the neighborhood or community, and the peer group were the major structures in which the individual lived, worked and played; once these structures were the source of most, if not all, of the emotional, financial, and status rewards individuals sought and received—no more. The family has moved away or been broken up by divorce; the neighborhood has been urban renewalized; individuals have moved to cities in search of work and a "better life." The unit of labor has become increasingly specialized; the organization of work increasingly larger, more impersonal, and less emotionally satisfying and stabilizing. With bureaucratization growing on every hand, it is only natural that unionization, the bureaucratic solution to settling working conditions, will rise.

5. *Erosion of middle class hegemony.* During the 1960s America heard, much to its surprise, that many Americans see little of value in the life style and attitudes of the Anglo-dominated middle class. Moreover, the institutions principally charged with preserving and perpetuating middle-class culture, such as the schools, military, churches, and public bureaucracies, either witnessed a dramatic decline in their social significance or a drastic reordering and redefinition of priorities (or both). Hospitals, which are run by, if not exclusively for, the middle class came in for a share of the abuse. The hiring of ethnic minorities, the new efforts at community relations, the relaxation of dress codes and styles of interpersonal behavior, among other programs of many hospitals, are examples of health care's reaction to the assertions of "counter cultures" by nonmiddle-class segments of the population. While the speed and tempo of the assault on middle-class culture and institutions has slackened, there is no retreat to the status quo ante; nor will there be one. Subcultures both within and outside the facility will continue to test the nerve, stamina, and good will of health care administrators.

## Hypotheses

In order to highlight the major empirical and theoretical findings of the present study, I have formulated the following hypotheses. These hypotheses are intended not to be taken as statements of fact, but rather as tentative conclusions which must be subjected to further testing and refining.

### GENERAL HYPOTHESES

1. Women and ethnic minorities are underrepresented in health care administration, especially in the top positions.
2. There is no significant representation of hospital or health care administration degrees among health care administrators.
3. Very few health care administrators come to their present position without previous administrative experience.

[ 176 ] **CONFLICT AND CONTROL IN HEALTH CARE ADMINISTRATION**

4. Individuals who hold administrative positions tend to rise vertically within the health industry rather than to enter it horizontally from other industries or professions.

   4a. Physicians and nurses are rarely found in administrative positions.

5. A high percent of health care administrators belong to professional associations and read trade publications and professional periodicals.

6. The profession is highly mobile, as illustrated by the high percent of administrators which reports a year or less in their present posts.

   6a. The high rate of personnel turnover in administrative posts is dysfunctional to the operations of the administrative system and dysfunctional for patient care.

7. Explaining work routines to and evaluating the performance of subordinates are the principal activities of health care administrators.

8. Administrators more frequently cite problems with subordinates than any other role partner.

9. While dealing with patients consumes little of the administrator's average day, a great majority of administrators report having problems with patients or their families.

   9a. Although they lack resources, patients are often either unwilling or unable to conform to the expectations and demands of health care workers and administrators, thus becoming a source of "problems" for the health care administrator.

10. Inadequate data and information and poor communications are problems shared by all health care administrators.

11. Rapidly changing and increasingly sophisticated medical and managerial technology and techniques are major sources of problems for health care administrators.

12. Organizations of health care workers are becoming increasingly aggressive role partners, with racism, sexism, and patients' rights joining economic and working conditions as common issues placed before administrators.

13. Physicians and medical staffs are sources of problems for all health care administrators.

13a. The resources held by medical staffs and physicians are becoming less valuable, and those of the administrator increasingly more valuable, to the health facility; thus there is an evolving role relationship underway.

14. Nurses are a common source of problems for health care administrators.

14a. Because many nurses reject their traditional exploitation and inferior role, the frequency of conflicts involving pay, privileges, and authority are expected to increase.

15. While boards of trustees and their equivalents are major links to political, social, and economic institutions, they are only slightly involved in the affairs of health care administrators.

15a. The closed decision-making and noninvolvement of health care workers, patients, and administrators in policy-making which characterizes the trustees/facility relationships suggests a strong parallel to the relationship between a community power structure and the masses of citizens.

16. Administrators see in-service training and continuing education as sources of information and skills which will allow them to do their job more successfully.

16a. Courses dealing with hospital administration, psychology and interpersonal relations, and the organization and methods of communications are the most frequently sought.

16b. These areas and topics closely parallel the activities and problems most frequently mentioned.

## OCCUPATIONAL PARTICULARITIES

17. Convalescent hospital administrators stand apart from administrators of general or extended care facilities.

17a. Convalescent hospital administrators report a lower frequency of college and postgraduate degrees.

17b. Convalescent hospital administrators tend to rise

within their sector rather than to enter it from other sectors of the health industry or the economy.

17c. Problems with patients or their families and with subordinates occupy the convalescent hospital administrator's time.

17d. The frequency with which convalescent hospital administrators mention or affirm problems with particular role partners suggest their resource-exchange pattern is not that of other health care administrators.

18. There are marked variations in the career patterns, activities, and problems with role partners among the three categories of administrators of general and extended care facilities.

18a. Chief administrative officers and administrative assistants have similar activity and problem profiles suggesting that there are some basic tasks common to administrative generalists within the health industry.

18b. Administrative generalists are more likely to report problems with trustees.

## SIZE AND TYPE OF FACILITY

19. Except for the time spent with patients, there is little difference in the average working day of the administrators of small (under 100 bed) and very large (700 and more bed) facilities.

20. The frequency with which administrators mention problems with particular role partners varies both with size and function of their facility.

20a. Among administrators of multifunction nonprofit hospitals and HMOs, size is related to variations in frequency of mentioning a problem and time spent with an activity.

20b. Proprietary, nonprofit, and government status is associated with variations in citing problems with role partners.

# NOTES

1. N. C. Bourestom and L. E. Gottesman, "Characteristics of Nursing Home Administrators and Quality of Care: Implications for Selection and Training," in M. J. Stott (ed.) *Education for Administration in Long Term Care Facilities* (Washington, D.C.: Association of University Programs in Hospital Administration, 1973), 101-111.

2. United States, DHEW, National Center for Health Statistics, "Selected Characteristics of Administrators for Nursing and Personal Care Homes: United States, June-August 1969," *Monthly Vital Statistics Reports* 20, supplement (14 January 1972), 1-9.

3. See S. H. Croog and D. F. Ver Steeg, "The Hospital as a Social System," in H. E. Freeman, S. Levine, and L. G. Reeder (eds.) *Handbook of Medical Sociology*, 2nd. ed. (Englewood Cliffs, N.J.: Prentice-Hall, 1972), 288-289.

# BIBLIOGRAPHY

*Health Care Administration:*
*Texts and Other General Sources*

Arnold, M. F., L. V. Blankenship, and J. M. Hess (eds.) *Administering Health Systems: Issues and Perspectives.* Chicago: Aldine, Atherton, 1971.

Brown, R. E. "Health Care Issues in the 1970s: Changing Management and Corporate Structure," *Hospitals* 44 (January 1970), 77-83.

Croog, S. H. and D. F. Ver Steeg. "The Hospital as a Social System," in H. E. Freeman, S. Levine, and L. G. Reeder (eds.) *Handbook of Medical Sociology,* 2nd. ed. Englewood Cliffs, N.J.: Prentice-Hall, 1972, 274-314.

Donabedian, A. *Aspects of Medical Care Administration: Specifying Requirements for Health Care.* Cambridge, Mass.: Harvard University Press, 1973.

Durbin, R. L. and W. H. Springhall. *Organization and Administration of Health Care: Theory, Practice, Environment.* St. Louis: C. V. Mosby, 1969.

Feldstein, M. S. *The Rising Cost of Hospital Care.* Washington, D.C.: Information Resources Press, 1971.

Friedson, Eliot (ed.) *The Hospital in Modern Society.* New York: Free Press, 1963.

–––. "Review Essay: Health Factories, the New Industrial Sociology," *Social Problems* 14 (1967), 493-500.

Georgopoulos, B. S. (ed.) *Organization Research on Health Institutions.* Ann Arbor: University of Michigan, Institute for Social Research, 1972.

Hanlon, J. J. *Principles of Public Health Administration,* 5th. ed. St. Louis: C. V. Mosby, 1969.

Heydebrand, W. V. *Hospital Bureaucracy: A Comparative Study of Organizations.* New York: Dunellen, 1973.

Levey, S. and N. P. Loomba. *Health Care Administration: A Selected Bibliography.* Philadelphia: J. B. Lippincott, 1973.

MacEachern, M. T. *Hospital Organization and Management.* Chicago: Physician's Record Company, 1957.

Moss, A. R. et al. *Hospital Policy Decisions: Process and Action.* New York: J. P. Putnam, 1966.

Owens, J. K. and R. K. Eisleben. *Modern Concepts of Hospital Administration.* Philadelphia: W. B. Saunders, 1962.

Penchansky, R. (ed.) *Health Services Administration: Policy Cases and the Case Method.* Cambridge, Mass.: Harvard University Press, 1968.

Perrow, C. "Hospitals: Technology, Structure, and Goals," in J. March (ed.) *Handbook of Organization.* Chicago: Rand McNally, 1965, 910-971.

White, P. E. and G. J. Vlasak (eds.) *Inter-Organizational Research in Health.* Washington, D.C.: Department of Health, Education and Welfare, 1971.

## Short Term General Care Hospital

Anderson, T. R. and S. Warkov. "Organization Size and Functional Complexity: A Study of Administration in Hospitals," *American Sociological Review,* 26 (1961), 23-28.

Argyris, C. *Diagnosing Human Relations in Organizations: A Case Study of a Hospital.* New Haven: Yale University, Labor and Management Center, 1965.

Bates, F. L. and R. F. White. "Differential Perceptions of Authority in Hospitals," *Journal of Health and Human Behavior* 2 (1961), 262-267.

Belknap, I. and J. Steinle. *The Community and Its Hospitals.* Syracuse, N.Y.: Syracuse University Press, 1963.

Bennis, W. et al. "Reference Groups and Loyalties in the Out-Patient Department," *Administrative Science Quarterly* 2 (1958), 481-500.

Brady, N. A. "The Corporate Hospital," *Hospitals* 44 (February 1970), 51-53.

Burling, T., E. M. Lentz, and R. N. Wilson. *The Give and Take in Hospitals.* New York: G. P. Putnam. 1956.

Duff, R. S. and A. B. Hollingshead. *Sickness and Society.* New York: Harper & Row, 1968.

Elling, R. H. "The Hospital-Support Game in Urban Center," in E. Friedson (ed.) *The Hospital in Modern Society.* New York: Free Press, 1963, 73-111.

Georgopoulos, B. S. (ed.) *Organization Research on Health Institutions.* Ann Arbor: University of Michigan, Institute for Social Research, 1972.

——— and F. C. Mann. *The Community General Hospital.* New York: Macmillan, 1962.

——— and A. Matejko. "The American General Hospital as a Complex Social System," *Health Services Research* 2 (Spring 1967), 76-112.

Ginzberg, E. *Urban Health Services: The Case of New York.* New York: Columbia University Press, 1971.

Gordon, P. J. "The Top Management Triangle in Voluntary Hospitals," *Journal of the Academy of Management* 4 (1961), 205-214.

Hanson, R. C. "Administrative Responsibilities in Large and Small Hospitals in a Metropolitan Community," *Journal of Health and Human Behavior* 2 (Fall 1961), 199-204.

Heydebrand, W. V. *Hospital Bureaucracy: A Comparative Study of Organization.* New York: Dunellen, 1973.

Jackson, L. G. *Hospital and Community.* New York: Macmillan, 1964.

Mayhew, B. H. and W. A. Rushing. "Occupational Structure of Community General Hospitals: The Harmonic Series Model," *Social Forces* 51 (March 1973), 455-461.

Perrow, C. "The Analysis of Goals in Complex Organizations," *American Sociological Review* 26 (1961), 854-866.

Pomrinse, D. S. "To What Degree are Hospitals Publically Accountable?" *Hospitals* 43 (1969), 41-44.

Ruchlin, H. S., D. D. Pointer, and L. L. Cannedy. "Administering Profit and Nonprofit Institutions," *Hospital Progress* 54 (October 1973), 67-69, 80.

Schwartz, J. L. "First National Survey of Free Medical Clinics, 1967-69," *HSMHA Health Reports* 86 (September 1971), 775-787.

Spitzer, W. O. "The Small General Hospital: Problems and Solutions," *Milbank Memorial Fund Quarterly* 48, Part 1 (October 1970), 413-447.

Starkweather, D. B. "Hospital Organizational Performance and Size," *Inquiry* 10 (November 1973), 10-18.

Steinwald, B. and D. Neuhauser. "The Role of the Proprietary Hospital," *Law and Contemporary Problems* 35 (Autumn 1970), 817-838.

Viguers, R. T. "Who's on Top? Who Knows?" *Modern Hospital* 86 (1956), 51-54.

Wilensky, H. L. "The Professionalization of Everyone?" *American Journal of Sociology* 70 (September 1964), 137-158.

Wren, G. R. "Administrators of Small Hospitals Have Same Motivating Factors as Those of Large, but Have Less Education and Experience," *Hospital Management* 3 (May 1971), 19.

Zald, M. N. and F. D. Hair. "The Social Control of General Hospitals," in B. S. Georgopoulos (ed.) *Organization Research on Health Institutions.* Ann Arbor: University of Michigan, Institute for Social Research, 1972, 51-81.

## Convalescent Hospital

Able, R. L. "Current Status of the Profession of Nursing Home Administration," *Journal of the American College of Nursing Home Administrators* 1 (Spring 1973), 3-10.

Bourestom, N. C. and L. E. Gottesman. "Characteristics of Nursing Home Administrators and Quality of Care: Implications for Selection and Training," in M. J. Stotts (ed.) *Education for Administration in Long Term Care Facilities.* Washington, D.C.: Association of University Programs in Hospital Administration, 1973, 101-111.

Earle, P. W. "The Nursing Home Industry," *Hospitals* 44 (1970), 45-51, 60-66.

Kaplan, J. "Nursing Home Administrative Training," *The Gerontologist* 9, 1 (1969), 70-71.

McCoy, L. "Licensing of Nursing Home Administrators," *Medical Care* 9 (March/April 1971), 127-135.

Meyers, D. D. "Practitioner's View of Education for Long-term Care Administrators," *Journal of the American College of Nursing Home Administrators* 1 (Winter 1972-73), 10-17.

Miller, D. B. *The Extended Care Facility: A Guide to Organization and Management.* New York: McGraw-Hill, 1969.

Reeder, L. G., D. H. Zimmerman, and E. B. Sheldon. "Improving Nursing Home Administration," *Journal of Health and Human Behavior* 4 (Spring 1963), 29-36.

Rogers, W. W. *General Administration in the Nursing Home.* Boston: Cahners, 1972.

Ruchlin, H. S. and S. Levey. "Planning for Long-term Care Administration Manpower: An Academic Perspective," in M. J. Stotts (ed.) *Education for Administration in Long Term Care Facilities.* Washington, D.C.: Association of University Programs in Hospital Administration, 1973, 24-38.

Stotts, M. J. (ed.) *Education for Administration in Long Term Care Facilities.* Washington, D.C.: Association of University Programs in Hospital Administration, 1973.

"Typical Administrator Relies on Experience, Not Classroom Work, HEW Survey Shows," *Modern Nursing Home* 28 (March 1972), 44, 74.

United States Department of Health, Education and Welfare, National Center for Health Statistics. "Selected Characteristics of Administrators for Nursing and Personal Care Homes: United States, June-August 1969," *Monthly Vital Statistics Reports* 20, Supplement (14 January 1972), 1-9.


## Mental Hospital

Ah, H. and S. Mailick. "Training for Mental Health Administrators," *Hospital and Community Psychiatry* 22 (November 1971), 348-352.

Belknap, I. *Human Problems of a State Mental Hospital.* New York: McGraw-Hill, 1956.

Caudill, W. *The Psychiatric Hospital as a Small Society.* Cambridge, Mass.: Harvard University Press, 1959.

Etzioni, A. "Authority Structure and Organizational Effectiveness," *Administrative Science Quarterly* 4 (1959), 43-67.

———. "Interpersonal and Structural Factors in the Study of Mental Hospitals," *Psychiatry* 23 (1960), 13-22.

Ewalt, J. P. *Mental Health Administration.* Springfield, Ill.: Charles C. Thomas, 1956.

Feldman, S. (ed.) *The Administration of Mental Health Services.* Springfield, Ill.: Charles C. Thomas, 1973.

Fuller, R. G. "A Study of Administration of State Psychiatric Services," *Mental Hygiene* 38 (April 1954), 117-235.

Hawkes, R. W. "The Role of the Psychiatric Administrator," *Administrative Science Quarterly* 6 (1961), 89-107.

Health, R. M. "The Role of Union and Management in Public Psychiatric Hospitals," *Journal of Mental Health Administration* 1 (Summer 1972), 15-22.

Henry, J. "The Formal Structure of a Psychiatric Hospital," *Psychiatry* 17 (May 1954), 139-151.

Heydebrand, W. V. *Hospital Bureaucracy: A Comparative Study of Organizations.* New York: Dunellen, 1973.

Lefton, M., S. Dinitz, and B. Pasamanick. "Decision-Making in a Mental Hospital: Real, Perceived, and Ideal," *American Sociological Review* 24 (December 1959), 822-829.

Squire, M. B. *Current Administrative Practices for Psychiatric Services.* Springfield, Ill.: Charles C. Thomas, 1970.

Stanton, A. H. and M. F. Schwartz. *The Mental Hospital.* New York: Basic Books, 1954.


## Labor Relations and Staff Organizations

Allen, A. D., Jr. "Systems View of Labor Negotiations," *Personnel Journal* 50 (February 1971), 103-114.

Alutto, J. A. "The Professional Association and Collective Bargaining: The Case of the American Nurses Association," in M. F. Arnold, L. V. Blankenship, and J. M. Hess (eds.) *Administering Health Systems: Issues and Perspectives.* Chicago: Aldine, Atherton, 1971, 103-126.

Argyris, C. *Diagnosing Human Relations in Organizations: A Case Study of a Hospital.* New Haven: Yale University, Labor and Management Center, 1965.

"Associate/Assistant Administrators Form Professional Groups: Health Care Management Association of Massachusetts," *Hospital Management* 3 (April 1971), 34.

Barnes, D. L. "Collective Bargaining for Radiologic Technologists," *Radiologic Technology* 45 (September/October 1973), 79-89.

Brown, R. E. "Health Care Issues in the 1970s: Changing Management and Corporate Structure," *Hospitals* 44 (January 1970), 77-83.

Bullough, B. "New Militancy in Nursing: Collective Bargaining Activities by Nurses in Perspective," *Nursing Forum* 10, 3 (1971), 273-288.

Clark, M. G. "The Organizations of Hospital Professionals," *Personnel* 47 (July/August 1970), 40-46.

Ehrenreich, B. and J. Ehrenreich. "Hospital Workers: A Case Study in the 'New Working Class,' " *Monthly Review* 24 (January 1973), 12-27.

Erickson, E. H. "Collective Bargaining: An Inappropriate Technique for Professionals," *Nursing Forum* 10, 3 (1971), 300-311.

Flowers, V. S. and C. L. Hughes. "Why Employees Stay," *Harvard Business Review* 51 (July/August 1973), 49-60.

Furrow, J. *AMA—Voice of American Medicine.* Baltimore: Johns Hopkins Press, 1963.

Grand, N. K. "Nursing Ideologies and Collective Bargaining," *Journal of Nursing Administration* 3 (March/April 1973), 29-32.

Gross, L., E. H. Grosof, and C. A. Yeracaris. "A General Theory of Labor Turnover in Hospitals," in E. G. Jaco (ed.) *Patients, Physicians and Illness. A Sourcebook in Behavioral Science and Health,* 2nd. ed. New York: Free Press, 1972, 343-353.

Health, R. M. "The Role of Union and Management in Public Psychiatric Hospitals," *Journal of Mental Health Administration* 1 (Summer 1972), 15-22.

Hiddle, A. J. and T. R. Covington. "American Society of Hospital Pharmacists View Collective Bargaining," *American Journal of Hospital Pharmacists* 30 (May 1973), 428-435.

Langer, E. "Inside the Hospital Workers: The Best Contract Anywhere," *New York Review of Books* 16 (20 May and 3 June 1971), 25-33; 30-37.

McKersie, R. B. and M. Brown. "Nonprofessional Hospital Workers and a Union Organizing Drive," *Quarterly Journal of Economics* (August 1963), 372-404.

Miller, J. D. and S. M. Shortell. "Hospital Unionization: A Study of the Trends," *Hospitals* 43 (1969), 67-73.

Miller, R. L. "Hospital-Union Relationship: Multi-Party Negotiations," *Hospitals* 45 (1 May and 16 May 1971), 49-54; 52-56.

Pointer, D. D. and H. Graham. "Recognition, Negotiation, and Work Stoppages in Hospitals," *Monthly Labor Review* 94 (May 1971), 54-58.

――― and N. Metzger. "Work Stoppages in the Hospital Industry: A Preliminary Profile and Analysis," *Hospital Administration* 19 (Spring 1972), 9-24.

Rakich, J. S. "Hospital Unionization: Causes and Effects," *Hospital Administration* 18 (Winter 1973), 7-18.

Schultz, R. and A. C. Johnson. "Conflict in Hospitals," *Hospital Administration* 16 (Summer 1971), 36-50.

Shinn, J. "How Local 1199 Wins Over Hospitals: Soul Power, Black Power, and $120.76 a Week," *Modern Hospital* 116 (January 1971), 39-42.

Van Cleve, W. J. "Collective Bargaining in the Health Care Industry," *Journal of the American Dietetic Association* 61 (December 1972), 633-636.

Wessen, A. F. "Hospital Ideology and Communication Between Ward Personnel," in E. G. Jaco (ed.) *Patients, Physicians, and Illness: A Sourcebook in Behavioral Science and Health.*, 2nd. ed. New York: Free Press, 1972, 325-342.

Wilensky, H. L. "The Professionalization of Everyone?" *American Journal of Sociology* 70 (September 1964), 137-158.

## Role Partners

### NURSES

Alexander, E. L. *Nursing Administration in the Hospital Health Care System.* St. Louis: C. V. Mosby, 1972.

Alutto, J. A. "The Professional Association and Collective Bargaining: The Case of the American Nursing Association," in M. F. Arnold, L. V. Blankenship, and J. M. Hess (eds.) *Administering Health Systems: Issues and Perspectives.* Chicago: Aldine, Atherton, 1971, 103-126.

Argyris, C. *Diagnosing Human Relations in Organizations: A Case Study of a Hospital.* New Haven: Yale University, Labor and Management Center, 1965.

Bullough, B. "New Militancy in Nursing: Collective Bargaining Activities by Nurses in Perspective," *Nursing Forum* 10, 3 (1971), 273-288.

Cleland, V. "Sex Discrimination: Nursing's Most Pervasive Problems," *American Journal of Nursing* (August 1971), 1542-1549.

Erickson, E. H. "Collective Bargaining: An Inappropriate Technique for Professionals," *Nursing Forum* 10, 3 (1971), 300-311.

Grand, N. K. "Nursing Ideologies and Collective Bargaining," *Journal of Nursing Administration* 3 (March/April 1973), 29-32.

Roberts, J. I. and T. M. Group. "The Women's Movement and Nursing," *Nursing Forum* 12, 3 (1973), 303-322.


### PHYSICIANS

Bates, F. L. and R. F. White. "Differential Perceptions of Authority in Hospitals," *Journal of Health and Human Behavior* 2 (1961), 262-267.

Becker, H. S. et al. *Boys in White.* Chicago: University of Chicago Press, 1961.

Brown, R. E. "In the Board-Administrator Relationships Hospital Tensions Threaten Tenure," *Modern Hospital* 73 (1949), 51-53.

Bugbee, G. "The Physician in the Hospital Organization," *New England Journal of Medicine* 261 (1959), 896-901.

———. "Administration and the Professional in the Hospital," *Hospital Administration* 6 (1961), 26-33.

Burling, T., E. M. Lentz, and R. N. Wilson. *The Give and Take in Hospitals.* New York: G. P. Putnam, 1956.

Coser, R. L. "Authority and Decision-making in a Hospital," *American Sociological Review* 23 (1958), 56-63.

Croog, S. H. and D. F. Ver Steeg. "The Hospital as a Social System," in H. E. Freeman, S. Levine, and L. G. Reeder (eds.) *Handbook of Medical Sociology,* 2nd. ed. Englewood Cliffs, N.J.: Prentice-Hall, 1972, 274-314.

"Doctors and Hospitals," *Modern Hospitals* 112 (January 1969), 69-98.

Dolson, M. "M.D.–Administrators Are Older, Earn More Money, Run Bigger Hospitals: Survey," *Modern Hospital* 112 (February 1969), 96-98.

Engels, G. V. "The Effect of Bureaucracy on the Professional Autonomy of Physicians," *Journal of Health and Social Behavior* 10 (March 1969), 30-40.

Gordon, P. J. "The Top Management Triangle in Voluntary Hospitals," *Journal of the Academy of Management* 4 (1961), 205-214.

Goss, M. E. W. "Patterns of Bureaucracy Among Hospital Staff Physicians," in E. Freidson (ed.) *The Hospital in Modern Society*. Glencoe: Free Press, 1963, 170-194.

Ludlam, J. E. "Physician-Hospital Relations: The Role of Staff Privileges," *Law and Contemporary Problems* 35 (Autumn 1970), 879-900.

Myerhoff, B. G. and W. R. Larson. "The Doctor as Culture Hero: The Routinization of Charisma," *Human Organization* 24 (Fall 1965), 187-191.

Roemer, M. I. and J. W. Friedman. *Doctors in Hospitals: Medical Staff Organization and Hospital Performance*. Baltimore: Johns Hopkins Press, 1971.

Smith, H. L. "Two Lines of Authority: The Hospital's Dilemma," in E. G. Jaco (ed.) *Patients, physicians, and Illness: A Sourcebook in Behavioral Science and Health*, 1st. ed. Glencoe: Free Press, 1958, 468-477.

Wilson, R. N. "The Physician's Changing Hospital Role," *Human Organization* 18 (Winter 1959-60), 177-183.

## BOARD OF TRUSTEES

Bellin, L. E. "Changing Composition of Voluntary Hospital Boards. An Inevitable Prospect for the 1970s," *HSMHA Health Reports* 86 (August 1971), 674-681.

Berger, I. and R. Earsy. "Occupations of Boston Hospital Board Members," *Inquiry* 10 (March 1973), 42-46.

Blankenship, L. V. and R. H. Elling. "Organizational Support and Community Power Structure," *Journal of Health and Human Behavior* 3 (1962), 257-269.

Brady, N. A. "The Corporate Hospital," *Hospitals* 44 (February 1970), 51-53.

Brown, R. E. "In the Board-Administrator Relationships Hospital Tensions Threaten Tenure," *Modern Hospital* 73 (1949), 51-53.

Elling, R. H. "The Hospital-Support Game in Urban Center," in E. Freidson (ed.) *The Hospital in Modern Society*. New York: Free Press, 1963, 73-111.

——— and O. J. Lee. "Formal Connections of Community Leadership to the Health System," *Milbank Memorial Fund Quarterly* 44 (July 1966), 294-306.

Goldberg, T. and R. Hemmelgarn. "Who Governs Hospitals?" *Hospitals* 45 (August 1971), 72-79.

Gordon, P. J. "The Top Management Triangle in Voluntary Hospitals," *Journal of the Academy of Management* 4 (1961), 205-214.

Hanson, R. C. "The Systemic Linkage Hypothesis and Role Consensus

Patterns in Hospital-Community Relations," *American Sociological Review* 27 (June 1962), 304-313.

Holloway, R. G., J. W. Artis, and W. E. Freeman. "The Participation Patterns of 'Economic Influentials' and Their Control of a Hospital Board of Trustees," *Journal of Health and Human Behavior* 4 (Summer 1963), 88-99.

Pfeffer, J. "Size, Composition, and Function of Hospital Boards of Directors: A Study of Organization-Environment Linkage," *Administrative Science Quarterly* 18 (September 1973), 349-364.

Viguers, R. T. "Who's on Top? Who Knows?" *Modern Hospitals* 86 (1956), 51-54.

Zald, M. N. "The Power and Function of Boards of Directors: A Theoretical Synthesis," *American Journal of Sociology* 75 (1969), 97-111.

## Consumer Participation

Barry, M. C. and C. G. Ships. "A New Model for Community Health Planning," *American Journal of Public Health* 59 (February 1969), 226-236.

Breslow, L. "Political Jurisdictions, Voluntarism and Health Planning," *American Journal of Public Health* 58 (July 1968), 1147-1153.

Brieland, D. "Community Advisory Boards and Maximum Feasible Participation," *American Journal of Public Health* 61 (February 1971), 292-296.

Croog, S. H. and D. F. Ver Steeg. "The Hospital as a Social System," in H. E. Freeman, S. Levine, and L. G. Reeder (eds.) *Handbook of Medical Sociology,* 2nd. ed. Englewood Cliffs, N.J.: Prentice-Hall, 1972, 274-314.

DuVall, W. L. "Consumer Participation in Health Planning," *Hospital Administration* 16 (Fall 1971), 35-49.

Hanson, R. C. "The Systemic Linkage Hypothesis and Role Consensus Patterns in Hospital-Community Relations," *American Sociological Review* 27 (June 1962), 304-313.

Howard, L. C. "Decentralization and Citizen Participation in Health Services," *Public Administration Review* 32 (October 1972), 701-717.

Jaeger, B. J. "Government and Hospital: A Perspective on Health Politics," *Hospital Administration* 17 (Winter 1972), 39-50.

Pomrinse, D. S. "To What Degree are Hospitals Publically Accountable?" *Hospitals* 43 (1969), 41-44.

Strauss, M. and I. deGroot. "Bookshelf on Community Planning in

Health," *American Journal of Public Health* 61 (April 1971), 656-679.

Wolfe, S. "Consumerism and Health Care," *Public Administration Review* 31 (September/October 1971), 528-536.

## Technology and Decision-Making

Andrews, C. T. *Financial and Statistical Reports for Administrative Decision-making in Hospitals.* Bloomington: Indiana University Press, 1968.

Berki, S. E. *Hospital Economics.* Lexington: Lexington Books, 1972.

Cloner, A. "The Influence of System Theory in Educating Health Service Administrators. The University of Southern California experience," *American Journal of Public Health* 60 (June 1970), 995-1005.

Coser, R. L. "Authority and Decision-making in a Hospital," *American Sociological Review* 23 (1958), 56-63.

Cronkhite, L. W., Jr. "Computer Brings Order to Clinical Scheduling Systems," *Hospitals* 43 (April 1969), 55-57.

DeMarco, R. M. "Planning a Computer for a Food Service Department," *Hospitals* 42 (May 1968), 107-113.

Donabedian, A. *Aspects of Medical Care Administration: Specifying Requirements for Health Care.* Cambridge, Mass.: Harvard University Press, 1973.

Emrich, R. and E. Zak. "Computer Assists in Utilization Review," *Hospitals* 42 (August 1968), 56-59.

Feldstein, P. J. "Applying Economic Concepts to Hospital Care," *Hospital Administration* 13 (Winter 1968), 68-69.

Grant, M. "Health Administration in the Computer Age," *Public Health Reports* 84 (May 1969), 409-414.

Greenwood, F. and C. R. Kendrick. "Computer Technology: A Challenge for Hospital Administrators," *Hospital Administration* 13 (Summer 1968), 62-67.

Gross, P. F. "Development and Implementation of Health Care Technology: The U.S. Experience," *Inquiry* 9 (June 1972), 34-48.

Haggerty, J. R. "Computerized Information Systems: Acceleration of Hospital Planning," *Hospitals* 44 (November 1970), 43-46.

Hardy, O. B. "Systematic Processes Applied to Health Care Planning," *Hospital Administration* 16 (Winter 1971), 7-24.

Keller, T. F. "The Hospital Information System," *Hospital Administration* 14 (Winter 1969), 40-50.

Ledley, R. S. "The Use of Electronic Computers in Medical Data

Processing Aids in Diagnosis, Current Information Retrieval and Medical Research Keeping," *I.R.E. Transactions on Medical Electronics* 7 (January 1970), 31-47.

Lefton, M., S. Dinitz, and B. Pasamanick. "Decision-making in a Mental Hospital: Real, Perceived, and Ideal," *American Sociological Review* 24 (December 1959), 822-829.

Mohr, L. B. "Organizational Technology and Organizational Structure: 13 Local Health Departments," *Administrative Science Quarterly* 16 (December 1971), 444-459.

Moon, J. E. "On-line Computer System is Memory for Patient Care Data," *Modern Hospital* 113 (July 1969), 70-72.

Moss, A. R. et al. *Hospital Policy Decisions: Process and Action.* New York: G. P. Putnam, 1966.

Packer, C. L. "Automation in the Personnel Department," *Hospitals* 45 (October 1971), 45-48.

Powers, A. M. and G. F. Whitlock, Jr. "Computerized Employee Data Aid Administrative Decision-making," *Hospitals* 42 (August 1968), 60-63.

Scott, W. R. "Professionals in Hospitals: Technology and the Organization of Work," in B. S. Georgopoulos (ed.) *Organization Research on Health Institutions.* Ann Arbor: University of Michigan, Institute for Social Research, 1972, 139-158.

Segal, M. "The High Cost of Hospitals," *Public Interest* 1 (Winter 1966), 39-54.

Somers, A. R. *Hospital Regulation: The Dilemma of Public Policy.* Princeton: Princeton University, Industrial Relations Section, 1969.

Souder, J. J. "Computers Can Bring a New Rationality into Hospital Design," *Modern Hospital* 110 (March 1968), 80-86.

Stout, W. J. "How the Systems Approach Aids Administrative Problem-solving," *Hospital Topics* 49 (November 1971), 42-48.

Truxal, J. G. "Technology and Health Services," *Proceedings of the IEEE* 57 (November 1969), 1802-1806.

Young, J. P. "A Conceptual Framework for Hospital Administrative Decision Systems," *Health Services Research* 3 (Summer 1968), 79-93.

## Education for Health Care Administrators

Ah, H. and S. Mailick. "Training for Mental Health Administrators," *Hospital and Community Psychiatry* 22 (November 1971), 348-352.

Arnold, M. F. "Education for Administration of Health Services," *Public Administration Review* 31 (September/October 1971), 537-542.

Bauerschmidt, A. D. "Calculus of Hospital Administration," *Hospital Administration* 16 (Fall 1971), 50-68.

Bourestom, N. C. and L. E. Gottesman. "Characteristics of Nursing Home Administrators and Quality of Care: Implications for Selection and Training," in M. J. Stotts (ed.) *Education for Administration in Long Term Care Facilities.* Washington, D.C.: Association of University Programs in Hospital Administration, 1973, 101-111.

Brown, R. E. (ed.) *Graduate Education for Hospital Administration.* Chicago: University of Chicago Press, 1959.

Cloner, A. "The Influence of System Theory in Educating Health Service Administrators. The University of Southern California Experience," *American Journal of Public Health* 60 (June 1970), 995-1005.

Gentry, J. T. et al. "Perceptual Differences of Administrators Regarding the Importance of Health Programs: Implications for Education for Health Services Administration," *American Journal of Public Health* 60 (June 1970), 1006-1017.

Griffith, J. R. "An Educational Challenge for the Programs and the Practitioners: The New Role of the Administrator," *Hospital Administration* 12 (1967), 127-142.

Hartman, G., S. Levey, and T. McCarthy. "The Impact of Graduate Programs in Hospital Administration," *Hospital Administration* 7 (Spring 1962), 45-47.

Kaplan, J. "Nursing Home Administrative Training," *The Gerontologist* 9, 1 (1969), 70-71.

Meyers, D. D. "Practitioner's View of Education for Long-term Care Administrators," *Journal of the American College of Nursing Home Administrators* 1 (Winter 1972-73), 10-17.

University of Michigan. *Education for Health Services Administration.* Ann Arbor: University of Michigan, 1972.

Motts, B. J. F. "The Crisis in Health Care: Problems of Policy and Administration," *Public Administration Review* 31 (September/October 1971), 501-507.

National Commission on Community Health Services. *Health is a Community Affair.* Cambridge, Mass.: Harvard University Press, 1966.

Raffel, M. W. "Education for Health Service Administration. Undergraduate Training for Health Administration," *American Journal of Public Health* 60 (June 1970), 982-987.

Roemer, M. I. "Changing Patterns of Health Services," *Annals of the American Academy of Political and Social Science* 346 (March 1963), 44-56.

———. "Education for Medical Care Administration," *Hospital Administration* 10 (Summer 1965), 6-18.

Ruchlin, H. S. and S. Levey. "Planning for Long-term Care Administration Manpower: An Academic Perspective," in M. J. Stotts (ed.) *Education for Administration in Long Term Care Facilities.* Washington, D.C.: Association of University Programs in Hospital Administration, 1973, 24-38.

Stotts, M. J. (ed.) *Education for Administration in Long Term Care Facilities.* Washington, D.C.: Association of University Programs in Hospital Administration, 1973.

Thompson, J. D. and G. L. Filerman. "Trends and Developments in Education for Hospital Administration," *Hospital Administration* 12 (1967), 13-32.

Weil, T. P. and W. J. Williams. "Training Health-Center Administrators: Some Alternatives," *New York State Journal of Medicine* 73 (1 February 1973), 475-484.

Westfall, R. "Educating for the Future," *Hospital Administration* 16 (1969), 81-94.

Ziegler, R. J. "Changing Characteristics of the Professional Program in Hospital Administration," *Personnel Journal* 50 (June 1971), 473-479.

## Studies of Health Care Administrators

Bauerschmidt, A. D. "Calculus of Hospital Administration," *Hospital Administration* 16 (Fall 1971), 50-68.

Bourestom, N. C. and L. E. Gottesman. "Characteristics of Nursing Home Administrators and Quality of Care: Implications for Selection and Training," in M. J. Stotts (ed.) *Education for Administration in Long Term Care Facilities.* Washington, D.C.: Association of University Programs in Hospital Administration, 1973, 101-111.

Connors, E. J. and J. C. Hutts. "How Administrators Spend Their Day," *Hospitals* 41 (February 1967), 45-50, 141.

Dolson, M. "Where Women Stand in Administration," *Modern Hospital* 108 (May 1967), 100-105.

———. "M.D.–Administrators Are Older, Earn More Money, Run Bigger Hospitals: Survey," *Modern Hospital* 112 (February 1969), 96-98.

———. "Administrators' Salaries, Education and Job Satisfaction Going Up, Study Shows," *Modern Nursing Home* 24 (May 1970), 57-60, 100.

———, R. F. White, and P. Van Ripper. "Study Reveals What Administrators Earn," *Modern Hospital* 106 (April 1966), 103-106.

Elling, R. H. and W. P. Shepard. "A Study of Public Health Careers: Hospital Administrators in Public Health," *American Journal of Public Health* 58 (May 1968), 918-924.

Gentry, J. T. et al. "Perceptual Differences of Administrators Regarding the Importance of Health Programs: Implications for Education for Health Services Administration," *American Journal of Public Health* 60 (June 1970), 1006-1017.

Hartman, G., S. Levey, and T. McCarthy. "The Impact of Graduate Programs in Hospital Administration," *Hospital Administration* 7 (Spring 1962), 45-47.

Lentz, E. M. "Hospital Administration—One of a Species," *Administrative Science Quarterly* 1 (1957), 444-463.

Letourneau, C. V. "Hospital Administration: A True Profession," *Hospital Administration* 13 (Winter 1968).

Metsch, J. M. "Professionalism in Administration," *Hospital Topics* 47 (September 1969), 50-53.

Murray, R. T., P. R. Donnelly, and M. Threadgould. "How Administrators Spend Their Time: A Research Report," *Hospital Progress* 49 (September 1968), 49-58.

Pecarchik, R. and W. G. Mather. "Lack of Business Skills Threatens Women Administrators," *Modern Nursing Homes* 24 (May 1979), 58.

Roemer, M. I. *Medical Care Administration: Content, Positions, and Training in the United States.* San Francisco: American Public Health Association, Western Branch, 1963.

Ruchlin, H. S. and S. Levey. "Planning for Long-term Care Administrative Manpower: An Academic Perspective," in M. J. Stotts (ed.) *Education for Administration in Long Term Care Facilities.* Washington, D.C.: Association of University Programs in Hospital Administration, 1973, 24-38

――― and D. D. Pointer. "Health Administration Manpower Research: A Critique and a Proposal," *Hospital Administration* 18 (Summer 1973), 81-104.

―――, ―――, and L. L. Cannedy. "Administering Profit and Nonprofit Institutions," *Hospital Progress* 54 (October 1973), 67-69, 80.

"Typical Administrator Relies on Experience, not Classroom Work, HEW Survey Shows," *Modern Nursing Home* 28 (March 1972), 44, 74.

Underwood, W. O. "A Hospital Director's Administrative Profile," *Hospital Administration* 8 (Fall 1963), 6-24.

United States Department of Health, Education and Welfare, National Center for Health Statistics. "Selected Characteristics of Administrators for Nursing and Personal Care Homes: United States, June-August 1969," *Monthly Vital Statistics Reports* 20 supplement (14 January 1972), 109.

Wesbury, S. A., Jr. "Career Patterns in Health and Hospital Administration," Ph.D. dissertation, University of Florida, 1972.

White, R. F. "The Hospital Administrator's Emerging Professional Role," in M. F. Arnold, L. V. Blankenship, and J. M. Hess (eds.) *Administering Health Systems: Issues and Perspectives.* Chicago: Aldine, Atherton, 1971, 51-69.

Wilensky, H. L. "Dynamics of Professionalism: The Case of Hospital Administration," *Hospital Administration* 7 (Spring 1962), 6-25.

"Womanpower in Hospital Administration," *FAH Review* 5 (August 1972).

Wren, G. R. "Administrators of Small Hospitals Have Same Motivating Factors as Those of Large, but Have Less Education and Experience," *Hospital Management* 3 (May 1971), 19.

## ABOUT THE AUTHOR

JERRY L. WEAVER is Associate Professor of Political Science, a faculty coordinator  of Health Care Administration at California State University, Long Beach. He received his Ph.D. in 1968 from the University of Pittsburgh. In addition to his interest in health care administration, Professor Weaver has conducted research on the health care needs of low income peoples and ethnic minorities. He is a member of the Executive Committee of the Committee on Health Politics, a body of political scientists interested in public policies in the area of health. Professor Weaver has published widely on Latin American comparative public administration and military as well as various aspects of health needs and public policy in the United States.